THE COMPLETE GUIDE TO CHAIR YOGA FOR SENIORS OVER 60

Low-impact Easy Exercises to Restore Strength, Mobility, Balance, and Lose Weight In 21 Days

TABLE OF CONTENTS

CHAPTER 8: CHAIR YOGA FOR MINDFULNESS AND RELAXATION   73

CHAPTER 9: CHAIR YOGA ROUTINES FOR SENIORS   83

Download the Video Exercises and 21-Day Challenge Tracker for Free!

Scan the QR code with your cell phone or ipad camera below:

INTRODUCTION

"We don't stop playing because we grow old; we grow old because we stop playing."
– George Bernard Shaw

George is a lively gentleman in his 60s who lives by the motto that age is just a number. Across the street lives his old college buddy, Ron, who often jokes that his best days are behind him and now it's just time to relax. George, on the other hand, sees retirement as a new chapter full of opportunities.

Every Saturday, George participates in a local softball league. He's often seen riding his bike, kite flying at the park, or organizing neighborhood scavenger hunts. His enthusiasm is infectious and he's known in the community for his playful spirit and zest for life.

Ron couldn't understand this enthusiasm for life because he was so preoccupied with "acting his age." He believed that growing older meant stepping back, settling down, and letting go of the playful activities he once enjoyed. He'd spend most of his days quietly reading the newspaper or watching television, occasionally peering out the window to see George zipping around the neighborhood on his bike.

One sunny afternoon, Ron's daughter and two young grandchildren came over for a visit. The kids begged Ron to play hide-and-seek with them in the backyard. At first, he hesitated, muttering something about "not being as spry as I used to be," but their eager smiles finally convinced him. After a few rounds, Ron realized he hadn't laughed this hard in years. He was out of breath and his knees ached, but the joy of playing with his grandkids was worth it.

That night, as he watched them curl up on the couch, still beaming from their games, he couldn't help but think about George's playful lifestyle. Maybe George had it right after all.

The next morning, he surprised everyone—including himself—by joining George on his morning bike ride. The wind in his hair and the warmth of the sun felt like a rush of youth. By the time they stopped for a rest, Ron was smiling wide. He finally understood the meaning behind the quote, "We don't stop playing because we grow old; we grow old because we stop playing."

From then on, Ron took every opportunity to be more playful, whether organizing family outings or joining George in the scavenger hunts. He realized that acting his age didn't mean giving up fun—it meant finding joy in living life to the fullest, no matter how old he got.

Perhaps Ron's story resonates with you. Maybe you've also felt the pressure to "act your age" to settle into a slower pace because that's what you believe is expected. Or perhaps it's not about acting your age at all. It could be that health challenges or physical limitations have made it difficult to stay active and find that sense of play again.

No matter the reason, this book was written to help you embrace the concept of playing and living life to the fullest. No one has to run marathons or climb mountains to recapture that sense of joy and vitality, and if that is your jam, kudos to you! I encourage you to keep at it safely, of course. If not, there's something more accessible that can help you reconnect with your body, boost your energy, and rediscover the simple pleasures of play—chair yoga.

Chair yoga offers a host of physical, mental, and emotional benefits that can transform your quality of life. Physically, chair yoga helps improve flexibility, strength, balance, and posture. Gentle stretches and poses keep muscles and joints active while strength-building exercises support better mobility and stability. Improved posture and alignment relieve tension and discomfort, making everyday activities more comfortable.

Mentally and emotionally, chair yoga provides valuable stress reduction, improves concentration, and fosters a deep sense of well-being. Breathing exercises calm the mind, while mindfulness practices help cultivate focus, making it easier to handle daily stressors. By releasing tension and enhancing inner awareness, chair yoga uplifts your mood and nurtures emotional balance.

Many seniors who have practiced chair yoga share inspiring testimonials about how it's positively changed their lives. Susan, in her late 70s, discovered that practicing just twice a week improved her posture and balance, giving her the confidence to navigate her neighborhood safely. Timothy, who once felt stiff and sluggish, admits that chair yoga brought a renewed sense of energy and clarity to his day, making him feel more youthful and vibrant. For Margaret, chair yoga is about finding calm amidst her busy family life. Deep breathing exercises help her sleep better and approach her days with a clear mind.

You can see similar results, but the best part is that these benefits will be related to you, your life, and what you value. This book will guide you to gaining the advantages of practicing chair yoga. Each chapter is carefully designed to build your confidence and comfort, whether you're new to exercise or have specific fitness goals in mind.

- In the first chapters, you'll find introductory information about chair yoga, including the basics of breathing and gentle poses to help you ease into the practice.
- Subsequent chapters will delve deeper into a range of poses for flexibility, strength, and balance, including adaptive options that can be modified to suit your mobility and fitness level.
- You'll also discover mindfulness practices and breathing techniques that complement the physical exercises, helping to deepen your connection to each movement.
- The final chapters offer full chair yoga sequences, guiding you step-by-step through complete practices, along with practical advice for incorporating these exercises into your daily routine.

Chair yoga offers gentle, seated movements that anyone can participate in, regardless of age or fitness level. The poses are designed to stretch your muscles, improve flexibility, and invigorate your mind. Through this practice, you'll find that even the smallest movements can spark a renewed connection with your body, releasing tension and inviting in more joy.

So, as you turn the page, be assured that you're stepping into a journey designed just for you. With chair yoga, you can reclaim your playful spirit and cultivate a lifestyle that energizes and inspires you. Embrace each breath and movement, and welcome the transformation that awaits!

CHAPTER 1

UNDERSTANDING THE PRACTICE OF CHAIR YOGA

"Yoga is not just repetition of few postures –
it is more about the exploration and discovery of the
subtle energies of life."

– Amit Ray

In her younger days, Gloria was a go-getter. She was the type of woman who thrived on having a packed schedule and didn't mind juggling responsibilities at work and at home. Whether she was organizing events, running errands, or volunteering in the community, Gloria's days were filled to the brim, and she loved it.

But as the years passed and she got older, her energy waned, and her body couldn't keep up with the fast pace she had once maintained effortlessly. The slow realization that she could no longer keep up left Gloria feeling anxious and unsettled. She struggled with the transition to a quieter lifestyle and began to experience waves of depression. Her restless energy had no outlet, and she felt adrift, unable to find purpose or satisfaction in her daily life.

During a routine doctor's visit, Gloria confided in her physician about her struggles. The doctor listened carefully and suggested trying chair yoga to help with her mental and physical well-being. Gloria was initially skeptical—could something as simple as chair yoga really make a difference? But she was willing to try anything that might offer some relief.

The first class was a bit awkward. Gloria felt stiff and uncertain in the poses. However, the soothing breathing exercises and gentle stretches gradually eased her tension. As she continued practicing, Gloria noticed that her joints felt more limber, her back pain lessened, and her posture improved. Yet, it wasn't just the physical benefits that kept her coming back. It was the way her restless energy shifted within her.

In each practice, she found herself focusing deeply on her breath and the simple yet precise movements, creating a calming rhythm that quieted her racing thoughts. The anxiety and sadness she'd felt slowly began to lift, replaced by a renewed sense of purpose and connection with her body. She started looking forward to her chair yoga sessions, where she could channel her once-boundless energy into mindful movement and breathing.

Over time, Gloria felt more grounded and empowered to explore new interests at a slower, more intentional pace. Chair yoga became her anchor, allowing her to tap into the subtle energy within and discover a new, fulfilling rhythm to life. She felt more at peace with herself, realizing that she didn't have to be in constant motion to find joy and purpose.

This chapter helps you connect with how chair yoga can help tap into your inner energy and how this can help you either find, rediscover, or strengthen your sense of purpose in this new stage of life.

Understanding Chair Yoga

With a long and detailed history, today, yoga is known worldwide as a holistic practice that blends physical exercises (asanas), breath control (pranayama), meditation, and ethical principles. With numerous styles like Ashtanga, Iyengar, Vinyasa, and chair yoga, it has become a practice that people of all ages can adapt to fit their individual needs.

This evolution has made yoga accessible to people seeking different benefits, whether it be increased flexibility and strength, stress reduction, or spiritual growth. Its centuries-old wisdom continues to offer a path toward harmony of body, mind, and spirit, enriching the lives of millions around the world.

In particular, chair yoga was developed as an accessible form of yoga specifically designed to accommodate individuals who face challenges with traditional mat-based yoga due to limited mobility, injury, or age-related physical changes. By using a sturdy chair for support, participants can perform modified yoga poses safely and comfortably while gaining many of the same physical and mental benefits as other yoga styles.

The practice of chair yoga gained popularity in the late 20th century when it became clear that more people could benefit from yoga if the physical barriers were reduced [4]. Teachers began adapting traditional poses to be performed while seated or using the chair for balance. The idea was to make yoga inclusive for those who couldn't participate in floor-based postures due to various health conditions, disabilities, or simply because they were new to yoga and needed extra stability.

Chair yoga includes poses that stretch and strengthen the body, as well as breathing exercises to calm the mind. It also focuses on improving posture and flexibility, areas that are particularly beneficial for older adults. Gentle twisting, bending, and lengthening movements help increase circulation, while breathwork (pranayama) promotes relaxation and mindfulness.

What makes chair yoga different from other styles is its emphasis on safety and support. Unlike more physically demanding forms of yoga, such as Ashtanga or Vinyasa, chair yoga allows for gradual progression and can be tailored to the needs of each individual. It's designed to provide a comprehensive workout without the need to get up or down from the floor, ensuring that people of varying fitness levels and abilities can practice.

This style is particularly popular in senior centers, rehabilitation facilities, and community classes. It empowers seniors to enjoy the benefits of yoga—such as improved strength, balance, and relaxation—without the risk of strain or injury. Ultimately, chair yoga fosters a welcoming environment where anyone can participate, cultivating both physical wellness and a deeper connection with one's body and breath.

Benefits of Chair Yoga for Seniors

Frank was an active and independent man in his late 50s who enjoyed tending to his garden, taking long walks in the park, and visiting his friends at the local community center. As he aged, however, he noticed a gradual decline in his muscle strength. Initially, it was subtle—he felt his knees ache more after gardening and his walks were shorter. Eventually, he struggled to rise from chairs without assistance and found it challenging to carry groceries into his home.

One day, while attempting to stand up after a social event, he lost his balance and fell, injuring his hip. The injury and his diminished muscle strength required him to rely on a walker and avoid strenuous activities. This sudden loss of independence took a toll on his spirit. He felt frustrated and embarrassed, needing help with simple tasks like showering or getting dressed. He stopped visiting the park and withdrew from friends, who he felt would see him as weak or incapable.

As Frank spent more time confined to his home, his energy levels plummeted. The once-vibrant man who loved sharing stories and laughter with his friends now found himself anxious and irritable. He felt powerless as if his body was betraying him, and the joy he once found in gardening and socializing had faded. This lack of activity further eroded his muscle strength, creating a vicious cycle that only deepened his feelings of helplessness.

Frank's reduced muscle strength not only took away his physical capabilities but also drained his energy and spirit. The loss of independence and the limitations he faced in daily activities left him feeling disconnected from his friends and hobbies, resulting in loneliness and depression. Without an outlet to nurture his body and mind, his sense of purpose waned, and he struggled to find the motivation to reconnect with the world outside his door.

There is still hope for someone like Frank because practicing chair yoga can help him regain muscle strength and, thus, allow him to maintain his independence, balance, and overall vitality. This benefit can be gained even with limited mobility or health concerns.

Building muscle strength involves activating the muscles and increasing muscle fiber size. During chair yoga, isometric contractions (where muscles tense without significant movement) and gentle weight-bearing exercises strengthen the muscles over time. For instance, standing poses supported by a chair engage the leg and core muscles, while seated arm raises and twists can tone the upper body. As muscles grow stronger, this improved muscle mass helps support bones, joints, and the cardiovascular system, reducing the risk of falls and injury.

Improved muscle strength is only one of the benefits that Frank will gain from practicing chair yoga [5]. More benefits include:

Increased flexibility

Increased flexibility is one of the primary benefits of chair yoga for seniors, contributing significantly to overall wellness. Gentle stretching movements help lengthen muscles, release tension, and maintain or improve joint mobility, enhancing daily life by allowing for greater ease and confidence in movement. Chair yoga helps counter the natural decline in muscle pliability and joint function due to aging by maintaining muscle pliability and joint function, enhancing blood flow, and loosening tight muscles and connective tissues.

Better Balance, Coordination, and Proprioception

Better balance, coordination, and proprioception (awareness of body position) reduce the risk of falls, allowing seniors to maintain independence. Chair yoga enhances these skills by encouraging gentle movements that strengthen muscles, improve spatial awareness, and promote a mindful connection between the body and mind. These exercises activate the brain's sensory and motor systems, strengthening muscles and improving communication between the brain and body, enhancing stability, spatial awareness, and energy balance.

Reduced Stress

As we grow older, stress can stem from health concerns, financial uncertainties, the loss of loved ones, or adjusting to retirement. Chair yoga reduces stress and cultivates inner calm through physical movement, mindful breathing, and relaxation techniques. Deep breathing exercises and gentle stretches activate the parasympathetic nervous system, reduce cortisol levels, and increase endorphin production, promoting a state of relaxation. This process also restores balance in the heart and solar plexus chakras, fostering emotional healing and personal power.

Better Sleep

Practicing chair yoga can help improve sleep quality, especially for seniors who may experience disturbances due to various reasons. Gentle stretches relieve muscle tension, and breathing exercises signal the body to relax, promoting better sleep by allowing the body to move into a restful state. Chair yoga also helps balance chakras, reducing anxiety and enhancing a sense of security and well-being, essential for cognitive function, immune health and emotional balance.

To supplement chair yoga, it is wise to also:

1. **Establish a bedtime routine:** Set aside at least 30 minutes to wind down before bed. Dim the lights, read a book, or listen to soothing music.
2. **Limit screen time:** The blue light from screens interferes with your body's natural sleep rhythms. Try to avoid screens at least an hour before bed.
3. **Create a comfortable sleep environment:** Ensure your mattress and pillows support your body well, and keep your room cool and quiet.
4. **Watch your diet:** Avoid large meals, caffeine, or alcohol too close to bedtime, as these can disrupt sleep.
5. **Stay active during the day:** Light exercise, like walking or swimming, can help regulate your sleep cycle.

Even when you feel your body winding down for the night, consider practicing some gentle chair yoga poses to help you drift off and wake up feeling your best. Your body and mind will thank you!

What to Expect From This Book

With an understanding of what chair yoga is and how it can help improve your quality of life, I say an official welcome to this chair yoga journey! I'm so glad you're here. I want you to be as energized as I am for the remaining steps of our continued journey together. So I am taking this time to give you a quick overview of what to expect from this book. We'll cover everything you need to start, even if this is your first time exploring yoga.

- **Introduction to Chair Yoga:** I'll guide you through setting up your space and choosing the right chair, and we'll discuss some important considerations before beginning.
- **Breathwork Basics:** Understanding the importance of breathwork will enhance your chair yoga practice immensely. I'll show you simple techniques to help control your breath and deepen your experience.
- **Warm-Up Exercises:** In this part of the book, we will focus on a few quick and gentle warm-up exercises that will prepare your body for deeper stretches and movements.
- **Chair Yoga Poses and Exercises:** We'll dive into a range of poses and exercises that focus on strength, mobility, stability, relaxation, and even weight loss.
- **Chair Yoga Routines:** I'll share some basic chair yoga routines that are easy to follow and designed to suit your specific needs.
- **21-Day Challenge:** I've included a complete 21-day challenge to help you establish a regular practice and see meaningful improvements over time.
- **Moving Beyond Chair Yoga:** Finally, I'll guide you on how to continue your journey, moving beyond chair yoga and improving your overall mental and physical health.

I'm excited to help you embrace this playful, enriching practice, no matter your age or experience level. So, settle into your chair and let's get started! The next chapter kickstarts your seated adventure as we'll dive into how to set up your space and prepare yourself for a rewarding chair yoga practice.

CHAPTER 2

GETTING STARTED WITH CHAIR YOGA

"In truth, yoga doesn't take time – it gives time."

– Ganga White

Anne was eager to experience all the wonderful benefits she'd heard about with chair yoga—more flexibility, less stress, and feeling better overall. But every time she thought about starting, she felt this hesitation settle in. The idea of a new routine seemed intimidating. What kind of chair should she use? Did she need any special equipment? Was she too out of shape to do it? The questions piled up, and as much as she wanted to dive in, she kept putting it off. There was always something else that needed her attention first and the uncertainty created resistance.

One morning, she woke up with a stiff back and tight shoulders after a night of poor sleep, and she realized she couldn't ignore it anymore. With determination, she cleared a space in her living room, picked out a sturdy chair, and found a simple, gentle routine to start with. She laughed at herself for being so nervous because, after just a few minutes of breathing and stretching, she already felt lighter and more at ease.

Anne's experience shows that it's normal to feel a little resistance when trying something new, but once you overcome that initial hesitation, you'll be amazed at how much more relaxed and vibrant you can feel. So, let's gently ease into it together, and soon, you'll find yourself moving through your chair yoga practice with joy and confidence.

What Do You Need for Chair Yoga?

Let's chat about what you need to get started with chair yoga! It's really simple, and you don't need much.

- **An Armless, Stable Chair:** The chair is the star of this practice, so make sure it's sturdy with no wobbling or uneven legs. Avoid chairs with arms, as they will get in the way of your stretches. A good dining chair or folding chair works well. Just check that the seat is firm enough to support you without sinking.
- **A Flat, Level Surface for Your Chair:** Find a solid, level surface to place your chair on. Hardwood floors or carpets work fine, but make sure your chair won't slide around too much. If your floor is slippery, consider placing a yoga mat under your chair for extra stability.
- **Flexible, Comfortable Clothing:** Wear something that won't restrict your movement. Opt for stretchy fabrics that aren't too tight or baggy. You don't want your clothes to catch or limit your stretches. Simple workout wear, like leggings or loose pants, and a breathable shirt should do the trick.
- **Space to Fully Extend Your Limbs:** Give yourself enough room to stretch your arms and legs without bumping into walls or furniture. Ideally, you'll need about an arm's length of space around your chair so that you can move freely.

It's that easy! Once you've got these basics set up, you'll be ready to sit down and flow into your practice comfortably and confidently.

Tips for Starting Chair Yoga

To ensure you stick with chair yoga, it is best to approach the practice with confidence and peace of mind. Here are a few tips to help you do just that.

Consult with Your Healthcare Professional

Before starting any new exercise routine, have a chat with your healthcare provider. Discuss your intentions and goals with them, and let them know of any medical conditions or physical concerns you have. They can offer specific advice or precautions tailored to your needs so you can practice safely.

Create a Safe and Comfortable Practice Space

Creating a yoga space that you genuinely want to use is key to making your chair yoga practice enjoyable. Rather than just plopping a chair down in the middle of the dining room, think of your practice space as a sanctuary—a dedicated corner that feels inviting and motivates you to show up.

- **Choose the Right Spot:** Find a corner or nook that offers peace and quiet, away from household distractions like TV noise or the buzz of daily activity. It could be a spot with a window that lets in natural light, a cozy corner with a view, or simply a well-ventilated area with fresh air.
- **Personal Touches:** Add a few items that inspire you. Maybe it's a calming plant or two, a small vase of flowers, or a cherished family photo that brings you joy. A favorite scented candle, essential oil diffuser, or soft blanket can also help create an environment that soothes your senses.
- **Music or Nature Sounds:** Soft background music or sounds of nature can enhance your experience. Create a playlist of soothing melodies, or let gentle birdsong or ocean waves play while you stretch and breathe.
- **Organize Props and Essentials:** Keep yoga props like cushions, straps, or a towel within arm's reach so you can easily access them when needed. Have a water bottle handy and consider a small basket for your phone or other personal items to stay organized.
- **Adjust Lighting:** Bright, harsh lighting can be distracting. Opt for natural light or soft lamps with adjustable dimmers to set the right mood for your practice, allowing your mind to settle and focus.

By designing a space that feels like a little retreat, you'll find yourself drawn to your chair yoga practice more often, helping you build consistency and fully enjoy each moment of gentle movement and mindful breathing.

Reflect on What Matters to You

Finding your "why" for doing chair yoga is like uncovering the heart of your practice. It's that deeper purpose that keeps you coming back to your chair day after day. To do so, think about what truly matters to you in your daily life and how chair yoga might support those priorities. Is it about staying active so you can spend more time playing with your grandchildren? Or maybe you want to ease tension and feel more peaceful throughout your day. Perhaps you're looking to reclaim a sense of strength and independence, or you simply want to move without pain.

Whatever your reasons are, focus on the core values or goals that will make a difference for you. Your why doesn't have to be complex—it can be as simple as "feeling less stressed" or "moving more freely."

By connecting with your why, you'll feel more inspired to practice because your efforts align with what matters to you. Your chair yoga routine will become a joyful ritual that nourishes your mind, body, and spirit in a meaningful way.

Set Realistic Goals

Setting goals is a crucial part of any fitness journey, including practicing chair yoga, because it gives you something to strive for and helps keep you motivated. Think of goals as your friendly guideposts—they give direction and support your purpose as you practice while letting you celebrate the progress you're making along the way.

Here's why it's important and how to do it in a way that excites you:

- **Clarity and Focus:** Goals help you figure out exactly what you want to achieve. Maybe it's improving your flexibility, reducing stress, or simply enjoying movement again. With a clear goal in mind, your practice becomes more intentional, and you can better measure your progress.
- **Breaking Big Goals into Smaller Steps:** A big goal might feel overwhelming at first. Let's say you want to feel more mobile overall. Instead of trying to overhaul everything all at once, break it down into smaller, manageable steps like "stretch for 10 minutes each day this week" or "work on improving my balance by holding

poses for a few extra seconds." These small wins add up and will motivate you to keep going.

- **Celebrate Milestones:** Recognize and celebrate each step forward, no matter how small it may seem. Perhaps you held a pose longer than before or noticed a new sense of calm after your session. Acknowledging your progress keeps the journey positive and encourages you to keep showing up.
- **Adapt and Adjust:** Life happens and your goals should be flexible enough to adapt to unexpected changes. If you miss a day or two of practice, don't be hard on yourself. Adjust your goals as needed and remember that consistency, not perfection, is key.

By setting goals that are realistic, meaningful, and achievable, you'll give yourself the gift of a practice that motivates you to roll out your mat, grab your chair, and breathe deeply. It's all about finding your rhythm and enjoying the journey at your own pace!

Listen to Your Body

When you're practicing chair yoga, it's crucial to listen to your body. Think of your body as a wise guide that gives you helpful feedback. Pay close attention to how you feel during each movement. If you notice that something doesn't feel right or a pose causes pain, stop immediately. It's better to modify or skip a pose than to push through discomfort and risk injury.

You can try smaller movements or reduce the range of motion if a stretch feels too intense. And if a pose just isn't working for you, that's perfectly okay. Your practice is about finding what feels good and safe for you, so don't compare your progress to anyone else's.

Over time, you'll find that your flexibility and strength will gradually improve, and poses that once seemed challenging will become easier. But be patient with yourself. The important thing is to approach your practice with kindness and curiosity, allowing your body to open up at its own pace. Your chair yoga journey is a personal one, and the more you listen to your body, the more you'll enjoy every gentle stretch and deep breath along the way.

Seek Professional Guidance

While this book is designed to help you get started on your own, if you're unsure about starting on your own, consider joining a chair yoga class or getting guidance from a certified instructor. They'll help you learn the poses correctly and ensure you're moving safely, especially if you have unique mobility concerns. Even an online video or book with clear instructions can help you build confidence.

Remember, chair yoga is all about finding gentle movement that works for your body and helps you feel your best. Be kind to yourself, take things at your own pace, and know that every little stretch and breath counts!

Common Misconceptions

It's completely normal to feel resistance when starting something new. Often, we shy away from new experiences because we believe the misinformation that's been spread around us. This isn't your fault—it's how our brains are wired. Our minds naturally prefer familiarity because it's safe and comfortable, a concept rooted in evolutionary biology. Our ancestors survived by sticking to known routines and avoiding risky situations that could threaten their survival.

However, while this protective instinct is useful in some situations, it can also keep us stuck in place when we want to embrace positive change. It's important to overcome this resistance, and one of the best ways to do that is to arm yourself with the truth.

Educate yourself by seeking accurate information from trusted sources or people who've been where you are now. Whether it's hearing from others who've tried the practice you're curious about or learning directly from experts in the field, filling your mind with knowledge will build your confidence and reduce that fear of the unknown. Here is my contribution to helping you sift through fact and fiction about chair yoga by debunking common misconceptions.

Misconception: It's only for seniors.

Truth: While chair yoga is fantastic for seniors or those with limited mobility, it's also beneficial for anyone who wants a little extra support in their practice. Office workers, those recovering from temporary injuries, and even seasoned yogis looking for a different way to stretch and strengthen can all benefit. The chair just adds another tool to your practice toolbox.

Misconception: It's too easy or not challenging.

Truth: Some people think chair yoga doesn't provide a "real" workout, but that couldn't be further from the truth. You can adjust the intensity to fit your fitness level, and even a gentle practice can be surprisingly effective for improving strength, balance, and flexibility.

Misconception: It has limited benefits.

Truth: It's easy to underestimate how powerful chair yoga can be. Besides being a low-impact form of physical activity, it offers comprehensive benefits like better muscle tone, reduced stress, improved flexibility, and greater mental clarity. It's not just "mild exercise"—it can help you feel revitalized inside and out.

Misconception: It's Only for the Inflexible or Physically Impaired

Truth: Although chair yoga is a wonderful option for those who find standing poses challenging, it's also great for those who want to focus on upper body strength or target specific muscle groups without the strain of traditional standing poses. It can be as gentle or as intensive as you like.

Misconception: It's Not 'Real' Yoga

Truth: There's a myth that because chair yoga involves a chair, it's not legitimate. But yoga is all about the mind-body connection, and you can fully achieve flexibility, strength, and mindfulness right there in your chair. Your practice doesn't need to look a certain way to be meaningful and effective.

No matter your age, experience, or mobility level, chair yoga can be adapted to suit your needs and help you feel better in your body. So, if you've been on the fence due to any of these misconceptions, know that the chair can be a versatile and supportive partner in your yoga journey! Starting something new is all about taking small, manageable steps. By understanding the truth, you'll empower yourself to break free from limiting beliefs and find the courage to give this new experience a shot. Once you do, you might be surprised at how rewarding and enriching it can be!

Your Mindset Going Into It

Your mindset plays a massive role in how you approach challenges, including chair yoga. With the right mindset, even moments that seem like failures become learning experiences that help you move forward with more wisdom. When you believe that you can grow and improve through effort and perseverance, it changes everything.

Take a moment to look back on your life experiences. Think about times when you faced challenges but pushed through despite the obstacles. Maybe it was a tough job that required resilience or a personal struggle that called for grit and patience. In those situations, it was your determination and inner drive that got you through.

Now, I want you to bring that same spirit to your chair yoga practice. Sure, there may be days when you don't feel like stretching or days when certain poses feel awkward, but each step forward brings you closer to a healthier, more flexible, and more confident you.

Remember, with every stretch, deep breath, and gentle movement, you'll discover a little more about your body's capabilities and your mind's potential. So, approach this practice with the understanding that progress doesn't have to be perfect; it's about being consistent and staying committed to your goals.

You've already proven that you have what it takes to overcome challenges, so keep that mindset and trust that you can succeed here, too. Here are some key mindset qualities to keep in mind as you prove to yourself that you can do this:

- **Openness to Adaptation:** Be willing to adapt poses and use props like the chair to make your practice accessible and safe. Making modifications doesn't devalue the benefits of yoga. They're simply a way to meet your body where it is right now and help you enjoy the practice more.

- **Patience and Self-Compassion:** Progress in yoga can be gradual, so treat yourself with kindness. Recognize your body's abilities and limitations without self-criticism. Celebrate small victories and give yourself credit for showing up, even if some poses take a little longer to master.
- **Focus on Breath and Mindfulness:** Concentrate on your breathing techniques and the mindful aspect of yoga. Deep, focused breathing enhances mental clarity, reduces stress, and helps you feel more present in each pose. We will expand on this in the next chapter.
- **Consistency Over Intensity:** Gentle, regular practice will bring more benefits than sporadic, intense sessions. Consistency helps build strength, flexibility, and mental resilience over time. Find a routine that works for you and stick with it, even if it's just a few minutes each day.
- **Mindfulness and Presence:** Approach yoga as a holistic practice that integrates physical, mental, and emotional health. It's not just about physical fitness but about creating space for yourself to find peace and balance.

By bringing these qualities into your mindset, you'll be better prepared to make the most of your chair yoga practice. You'll find joy in the journey as you connect more deeply with yourself and embrace this playful, gentle way of staying active.

With this mindset in place, let's move forward to the next chapter and explore the breathing exercises that will enhance your chair yoga practice.

CHAPTER 3

BREATHING TECHNIQUES

"No matter what we eat, how much we exercise, how resilient our genes are, how skinny or young or wise we are-none of it will matter unless we're breathing correctly."

– James Nestor

Karen had always prided herself on being strong, but she didn't realize just how stressed she was as she navigated life as a senior until she had a panic attack one evening. Her heart was racing, her breath came in shallow, quick bursts, and she felt completely overwhelmed. It wasn't until later, reflecting on that experience, that she recognized she often breathed that way—short, rapid breaths that barely filled her lungs. She hadn't noticed how much this breathing pattern mirrored her anxiety and contributed to her stress.

When Karen began chair yoga, she became more aware of her breathing patterns and what they represented. Through the gentle stretches and movements, she practiced inhaling deeply and exhaling slowly, and soon, she noticed something remarkable: this intentional breathing brought her a sense of calm she hadn't felt in years.

It was a beautiful, cyclic effect. As she learned to control her breath during her chair yoga sessions, she found that she could bring the same focus and steadiness to her daily life. Whenever she felt stress creeping in, she would pause, close her eyes, and breathe deeply. The slow, rhythmic breaths grounded her and helped her navigate difficult moments with more ease.

This newfound awareness didn't just transform her yoga practice. It became a vital tool that allowed Karen to handle stress more effectively and regain her inner balance. She realized that breathwork was more than just an exercise—it was her anchor in a busy, unpredictable world. This is a universal truth that applies to all of us and this chapter helps you make great use of this tool.

Pranayama (Breath Control)

In the world of yoga, breath represents so much more than just a physical function. It's the very essence of life itself, known as prana or life force, in Sanskrit. When you breathe deeply and fully, you're not just taking in oxygen—you're inviting a flow of energy that connects your body and mind.

Think of your breath as your inner rhythm that guides each movement and moment, both on and off the mat. Or in this case, on and off your chair. In yoga, breath is like a bridge between the physical and the mental. It's the tool that can help you ground yourself when you're anxious or feeling scattered, or energize you when you're tired and in need of a boost. Every inhale brings in new energy, while every exhale releases tension and makes space for peace.

Breathwork, also called pranayama, is a practice of consciously controlling your breath to promote relaxation, clarity, and vitality [6]. It's a way to cultivate a state of calm in the mind while keeping the body steady and present. No matter where you are in your yoga journey, your breath is your constant companion—a gentle reminder to slow down, find balance, and be fully present in the moment.

So, as you move through your chair yoga practice, treat your breath as a guiding force. Feel its rhythm, and let it carry you toward a deeper connection with yourself and the world around you. Additional benefits to be experienced include:

- **Reduces Stress and Keeps You Calm:** Deep breathing activates the parasympathetic nervous system, which triggers your body's relaxation response. When you take slow, full breaths, you send a message to your brain to calm down, which then relaxes your whole body. You'll notice your shoulders drop, your muscles loosen, and your mind feels more at ease.
- **Increases Energy Levels:** Shallow breathing means less oxygen, which leaves you feeling sluggish. With breathwork, you draw in more oxygen, which circulates to your brain and muscles, giving you a natural boost of energy. If you feel more alert and clear-headed after a deep breathing session, that's your body recharging itself.
- **Boosts Immunity:** Oxygen plays a role in maintaining a strong immune system. Deep breathing encourages better circulation, helping oxygen and nutrients reach your cells while also eliminating toxins. If you notice you're catching fewer colds or generally feeling healthier, breathwork might be one reason.
- **Relieves Pain:** Deep breaths prompt the release of endorphins, your body's natural painkillers. These feel-good chemicals help alleviate discomfort and reduce tension. Whether it's easing a headache or soothing stiff joints, you may find breathwork lessens pain naturally.
- **Lowers Blood Pressure:** Slow, controlled breathing reduces the levels of cortisol, the stress hormone, in your body. This leads to lower blood pressure and a healthier heart. Over time, you may notice your blood pressure readings improving as you practice consistent breathwork.

Every so often, simply take a moment to breathe slowly and intentionally. Notice how your body feels afterward. Do you sense that peaceful calm, that boost of energy, or maybe just a lighter, happier mood? These signs let you know you're reaping the benefits of this simple yet powerful practice.

Simple Breathing Exercises

Consciously controlling your breath can be done in several ways. In this section, we will explore three of them.

Diaphragmatic Breathing

Diaphragmatic breathing, also known as belly breathing, is one of the simplest and most effective ways to enhance your chair yoga practice—and your daily life [7]. It's all about using your diaphragm, the large muscle located just below your lungs, to take deep, full breaths.

The diaphragm is the primary muscle used for breathing. As you practice this technique, the diaphragm becomes more efficient at pulling air into your lungs, which increases the supply of oxygen to your body.

When you breathe deeply and fully engage your diaphragm, your lungs expand completely, allowing you to take in more oxygen than shallow breathing can. This surge of oxygen gets distributed to every cell, tissue, and organ in your body, improving cellular function and overall vitality.

The increased oxygen supply also positively impacts the nervous system. Deep, diaphragmatic breaths activate the parasympathetic nervous system to counteract the effects of stress hormones like cortisol. This switch induces a calming effect, helping to lower your heart rate, reduce blood pressure, and ease muscle tension.

Additionally, this type of breathing promotes mental clarity and emotional balance, as it encourages you to focus inward and become more mindful of your body's natural rhythms. Over time, diaphragmatic breathing can significantly reduce anxiety and promote a lasting sense of calm and relaxation.

When you practice diaphragmatic breathing, you allow your belly to expand as you inhale and naturally contract as you exhale. This way of breathing helps you engage the diaphragm fully, allowing your lungs to fill up with air and ensuring a steady flow of oxygen into your body.

Here's how to try it:

1. **Find a Comfortable Position:** Sit in your chair with your feet flat on the ground, or lie down if that's more comfortable. If sitting, ensure that your back is straight.
2. **Place Your Hands on Your Belly:** Gently rest one hand on your chest and the other on your belly so you can feel how your body moves with each breath.
3. **Inhale Deeply Through Your Nose:** As you breathe in, let your belly rise and expand, pushing your hand out. Imagine filling your abdomen with air like a balloon. During this movement, your chest should remain still.

4. **Exhale Slowly Through Your Mouth:** As you breathe out, feel your belly slowly deflate. Ensure this breath is released through pursed lips as if you are whistling. Your chest should remain mostly still while your diaphragm does the work.
5. **Repeat.** Do Steps 1 to 4 for 2 to 4 minutes to start.

Practicing this breathing technique is a great exercise before starting your chair yoga routine, or you can simply do it anytime during the day when you feel overwhelmed or anxious.

Incorporate diaphragmatic breathing into your chair yoga sessions by using it with gentle stretches or relaxation poses. Deep breaths will help you settle into poses, relax your muscles, and focus your mind.

In daily life, it can be practiced while reading, walking, or even watching TV. It's particularly helpful in the evening to unwind before bed. Start with just a few minutes and work your way up—your breath will become a reliable companion to help you stay grounded and energized.

Equal Breathing

Equal breathing, or sama vritti in Sanskrit, is a simple yet powerful breathing technique that can help you reduce stress and improve focus [8]. The idea is to match the length of your inhale with your exhale, creating a balanced, steady rhythm. It's a wonderful tool to calm the mind and balance the respiratory system.

To practice equal breathing:

1. **Find a Comfortable Position:** Sit up straight in your chair with your feet firmly on the ground, or lie down if that's more comfortable. Close your eyes.
2. **Take a Deep Breath:** Inhale deeply through your nose, filling your lungs, and count the number of seconds it takes to complete your inhale. Try to reach a count of four to start.
3. **Hold Your Breath:** Do this for a count of one.
4. **Exhale for the Same Count as You Inhaled:** Slowly exhale through your nose for the same number of seconds as you inhale. If you took four seconds to breathe in, take four seconds to breathe out.

5. **Repeat:** Continue this pattern for several minutes, finding a steady, even pace. Gradually increase the duration of your inhales and exhales.

There are many benefits of equal breathing. The first of this list is reduced stress and improved focus. By slowing down and balancing your breathing, you activate the parasympathetic nervous system, helping you relax and stay calm. The rhythmic pattern also quiets your mind and helps you focus better.

Another huge benefit is that the practice balances the respiratory system by ensuring that your lungs are functioning effectively. It also gently massages your diaphragm, strengthening your respiratory system over time.

You can incorporate this technique into your chair yoga practice as a warm-up before starting your poses or use it during meditation for deeper concentration. It's also helpful in daily life when you need to center yourself, such as before a challenging conversation or after a long day. Practicing it before bed can prepare your body and mind for restful sleep.

Incorporating equal breathing into your routine will help you find balance, soothe your nerves, and face life's challenges with a clear mind. Start with just a few minutes and work your way up, letting your breath guide you toward calm and steady well-being.

Pursed Lip Breathing

Pursed lip breathing helps you control your breath and keep your airways open for longer [9]. The technique is especially helpful if you ever feel short of breath or find yourself breathing too quickly. The method involves breathing out through tightly pressed lips to slow down the exhalation using these steps:

1. **Find a Comfortable Position:** Sit down with your feet flat on the ground or lie down if that's more comfortable. Keep your shoulders relaxed.
2. **Inhale Through Your Nose:** Take a slow, deep breath through your nose, letting your belly expand as you breathe in. Do this for at least two seconds.
3. **Purse Your Lips:** Pucker your lips as if you're going to whistle or blow on hot food.

4. **Exhale Through Your Lips:** Breathe out slowly through your pursed lips for about twice as long as you inhaled. If you inhaled for two seconds, aim to exhale for four seconds.
5. **Repeat:** Continue this pattern for a few minutes, gradually easing into a rhythm that feels relaxing and natural.

You can expect the following benefits from practicing pursed lip breathing:

- **Controls Breathing:** By slowing down your exhalation, you can control your breathing and take in more air with each breath.
- **Keeps Airways Open Longer:** The pressure created by pursed lips helps keep the airways open, preventing them from collapsing and making breathing easier.
- **Relaxes Air Passages:** It allows you to gently relax the muscles around your airways, which is especially useful if you're experiencing shortness of breath or tightness.

Incorporate pursed lip breathing into your chair yoga sessions to help you ease into deep stretches or relaxation poses. It's also great for managing your breath during stressful moments or after physical activity. Practice it throughout your day, particularly if you feel out of breath or need a calming reset.

Make this technique part of your daily routine, and you'll notice yourself breathing more deeply and comfortably. It will help you feel in control of your breath and calm your nerves, no matter what challenges the day brings.

With these breathing techniques in your toolkit, let's move on to the next chapter and explore how to gently prepare your body for a fulfilling chair yoga practice.

CHAPTER 4

PREPARING THE BODY FOR CHAIR YOGA

"The nature of yoga is to shine the light of awareness into the darkest corners of the body."

– Jason Crandell

Paul was eager to start chair yoga after hearing about its incredible benefits, so he jumped straight into his first session without much thought. He stretched deeply and tried to keep up with all the poses, but he ended up feeling stiff and unhappy. A little research showed him that his sore muscles were the result of not preparing properly.

When he approached his next chair yoga session, he took a different approach. He spent a few minutes warming up, moving his joints gently and preparing his muscles for deeper stretches. This time, he was more mindful of his limits and eased into the poses instead of forcing himself too far.

As a result, he felt energized and more relaxed after the session, with none of the soreness he experienced before. Preparing his body had made all the difference.

This chapter will help you avoid Paul's mistakes by showing you how to gently warm up and prepare for your chair yoga practice. With a little preparation, you'll find each session more enjoyable and rewarding!

Why Warming Up Is Necessary

Warming up before chair yoga is like slowly easing your body into a gentle embrace. It prepares your muscles, joints, and mind for the movements to come, helping to unlock tension and stiffness that naturally build up over time. Think of it like this: just as you wouldn't jump straight into a pool without dipping your toes in first, you shouldn't dive into yoga without gradually warming up.

Warming up matters! Here are some of the reasons why:

1. **Increases Blood Flow:** Warming up encourages blood flow to your muscles, which helps them loosen and makes stretching easier and safer.
2. **Lubricates Your Joints:** Gentle, circular movements and light stretches help stimulate the production of synovial fluid around your joints, making them more flexible and less prone to stiffness.
3. **Reduces Injury Risk:** Preparing your body with a warm-up reduces the risk of injury by making your muscles more pliable and your movements more controlled.
4. **Enhances Mind-Body Connection:** It allows you to tune into how your body feels before you begin, so you're more aware of your limits and better equipped to adapt the poses to your comfort level.
5. **Calms Your Mind:** Warming up gives you a moment to breathe deeply and let go of distractions, helping you to enter the session with a clear and focused mind.

Make sure to give yourself a few minutes to gently wake up your body before each chair yoga session. You'll find that the poses feel smoother, your muscles respond better, and your whole practice becomes a more pleasant experience!

Tips for Effective Warmups

Here are some practical tips to help you get the most out of your warm-up:

1. **Start Slow and Gentle:** Begin with light stretches that don't require much range of motion. Think of simple neck rolls, shoulder shrugs, or gentle twists to ease your body into the routine.
2. **Breathe Deeply:** Deep, controlled breathing not only calms your nerves but also brings more oxygen to your muscles. Inhale through your nose and exhale through your mouth, matching your breath with each movement.
3. **Focus on Problem Areas:** If you tend to feel tightness in certain areas (like your neck, shoulders, or lower back), give them extra attention during your warm-up. Spend a little more time stretching these muscles to help loosen them up.
4. **Stay Within Your Comfort Zone:** Don't push too hard right away. Listen to your body, and if a particular movement feels uncomfortable or painful, ease off and modify the stretch. Variations are provided with the warmup exercises that will be outlined below.
5. **Gradually Increase Intensity:** As your muscles warm up and your range of motion improves, you can deepen the stretches a bit more. Just be mindful of staying relaxed and avoiding sudden, jerky movements.
6. **Create a Routine:** Consistency is key to reaping the benefits of a warm-up. Find stretches that work best for you and turn them into a familiar routine before each session.
7. **Enjoy the Process:** Warming up should feel good and relaxing. Use it as an opportunity to clear your mind, set intentions for your practice, and connect with your body.

These tips will help ensure that your muscles are ready to engage fully, reducing the risk of strain while making your chair yoga session more enjoyable and effective.

Warmup Exercises

You don't have to reinvent the wheel when warming up. Luckily, just like with the chair yoga poses, there are a variety of exercises that have already been established to yield great results to choose from. Let's go through some of these now.

Neck Stretches

Neck Rotation and Neck Massage

- Reduces tension

- Improves circulation
- Relieves stress

Instructions for Neck Rotation:

1. Sit comfortably in your chair, keeping your back straight and feet flat on the floor.
2. Start by lowering your chin toward your chest, feeling a gentle stretch in the back of your neck.
3. Slowly rotate your head to the right, drawing a small circle with your chin.
4. Bring your head back and around to the left, completing a full circle.
5. Repeat in this direction 3-5 times, then reverse direction.

Instructions for Neck Massage:

1. Sit comfortably with your back straight and feet flat on the floor.
2. Place your fingertips on the base of your skull, on either side of your spine.
3. Apply gentle pressure with your fingertips, massaging in small circles down to your shoulders.
4. Gradually work your way up and down your neck, adjusting pressure as needed.

Neck Bends Left and Right

- Relieves stiffness
- Increases flexibility
- Reduces headaches

Instructions for Neck Bends Left and Right:

1. Sit up straight in your chair with your feet flat on the floor and your shoulders relaxed.
2. Take a deep breath, and on the exhale, slowly bend your head to the right, bringing your right ear closer to your right shoulder.
3. Hold the stretch for a few seconds, feeling the stretch along the left side of your neck. Keep your shoulders relaxed. Avoid tilting them.
4. Slowly return to the starting position, then repeat the same motion on the left side, bringing your left ear closer to your left shoulder.

5. Repeat the bend to each side 3-5 times.

Shoulder Rolls

- Loosens tension
- Improves posture
- Increases blood flow

Instructions for Shoulder Rolls:

1. Sit comfortably with your feet flat on the floor and your spine straight.
2. Let your arms hang by your sides and keep your shoulders relaxed.
3. Inhale deeply, and on the exhale, lift your shoulders toward your ears.
4. Roll your shoulders backward in a circular motion, squeezing your shoulder blades together and opening up your chest.
5. Complete the circle by bringing your shoulders down and forward, then back up to your ears again.
6. Repeat this motion 5-10 times, focusing on smooth, controlled movements.
7. Switch direction by rolling your shoulders forward for another 5-10 times.

Upper Body Warm-Up

Seated Tadasana

- Improves posture
- Grounds your energy for focus and relaxation
- Increases self-awareness

Instructions for Seated Tadasana:

1. Sit in your chair with your feet flat on the ground, knees at a 90-degree angle, and spine straight.
2. Place your hands on your thighs, or let them hang by your sides.
3. Engage your core muscles gently, drawing your belly button toward your spine to support your lower back.

4. Lift your chest and roll your shoulders back and down, keeping your chin parallel to the floor.
5. Imagine a string gently pulling the top of your head toward the ceiling, lengthening your spine.
6. Close your eyes if you like, and take a few deep breaths, feeling the steady alignment from your hips to your head.

Arm Stretches

- Releases tension
- Increases flexibility
- Boosts circulation

Instructions for Arm Stretches:

1. Sit up straight in your chair with your feet flat on the ground and your shoulders relaxed.
2. Inhale deeply, and as you exhale, reach your right arm straight up toward the ceiling. Hold it for a moment, feeling the stretch along your side.
3. Bring your right arm down, and repeat on the left side, reaching straight up.
4. After stretching each arm individually, reach both arms straight up together, interlacing your fingers if possible.
5. Lean gently to the right to stretch your left side, then come back to the center and lean to the left to stretch your right side.
6. Relax your arms by your sides, and roll your shoulders a couple of times to release any lingering tension.

Arm Lifts

- Improves mobility
- Improves posture
- Boosts circulation

Instructions for Arm Lifts:

1. Sit comfortably in your chair with your back straight and feet flat on the floor.

2. Let your arms hang naturally by your sides.
3. Inhale deeply, and as you exhale, lift your right arm straight up toward the ceiling, keeping it close to your ear.
4. Hold your arm up for a few seconds while feeling the stretch down your side, then gently bring it back down on the next exhale.
5. Repeat with your left arm, lifting it straight up and holding it for a few seconds.
6. Continue alternating between both arms, lifting each one 3-5 times.

Arm Circles

- Relieves stiffness
- Improves flexibility
- Improves circulation

Instructions for Arm Circles:

1. Sit or stand with your back straight, keeping your shoulders relaxed and feet firmly on the floor.
2. Extend your arms to the sides so they're parallel to the ground, with palms facing down.
3. Start making small circles in the air with your fingertips. Move slowly at first to warm up your shoulder joints.
4. Gradually increase the size of your circles while maintaining controlled movements. Breathe steadily as you circle your arms.
5. After about 10-15 seconds, reverse direction and start circling your arms the other way, again starting with small circles and building up.
6. Repeat 2-3 sets of circles in both directions.

Seated Torso Circles

- Loosens tight muscles
- Engages core muscles
- Increases flexibility

Instructions for Seated Torso Circles:

1. Sit comfortably on the edge of your chair with your feet flat on the ground, about hip-width apart.

2. Place your hands on your thighs or knees for support and keep your spine straight.
3. Inhale deeply, and as you exhale, lean forward and to the right, moving your torso in a circular motion.
4. Circle your torso to the back, then to the left, and finally to the front to complete the circle.
5. Move gently, focusing on stretching each part of your core and lower back as you circle around.
6. Repeat the circular motion 5-10 times, then switch directions and circle the opposite way.

Shoulder Blade Squeezes

- Releases tension
- Improves posture
- Opens the chest

Instructions for Shoulder Blade Squeezes:

1. Sit comfortably in your chair with your back straight and feet flat on the floor.
2. Let your arms hang down naturally by your sides.
3. Inhale deeply, and as you exhale, draw your shoulder blades together as if you're trying to hold a pencil between them.
4. Keep your neck relaxed and avoid raising your shoulders to your ears.
5. Hold the squeeze for 3-5 seconds, then release your shoulder blades back to a neutral position.
6. Repeat this movement 8-10 times, breathing steadily throughout the exercise.

Warmup The Lower Body and Back

Seated Marches

- Warms up leg muscles
- Increases blood flow
- Improvs balance

Instructions for Seated Marches:

1. Sit comfortably on the edge of your chair with your feet flat on the ground and your back straight.

2. Place your hands on the sides of the chair for support.
3. Inhale deeply, and as you exhale, lift your right knee toward your chest to create a 90-degree angle at your hip.
4. Lower your right leg back down and lift your left knee in the same way, just like you're marching.
5. Continue alternating legs in a steady rhythm, lifting each knee for 1-2 seconds before switching sides.
6. Repeat this for about 30 seconds to a minute, moving as smoothly and steadily as possible.

Leg Lifts

- Strengthens leg muscles
- Improves circulation
- Improves balance

Instructions for Leg Lifts:

1. Sit up straight in your chair with your feet flat on the ground and your hands resting on the sides of the chair.
2. Inhale deeply, and as you exhale, lift your right leg in front of you so that it's parallel to the floor. Your knee should stay straight as you lift.
3. Hold your leg in this lifted position for 1-2 seconds, then lower it back down gently.
4. Repeat the same movement with your left leg, lifting it until it's parallel to the floor.
5. Alternate between legs for about 8-10 lifts per side, moving in a steady rhythm while keeping your core engaged.

Knee Lifts

- Engages core muscles
- Improves circulation
- Enhances coordination

Instructions for Knee Lifts:

1. Sit comfortably in your chair with your feet flat on the ground and your back straight.
2. Rest your hands on your thighs or the sides of your chair for support.

3. Inhale deeply, and as you exhale, lift your right knee toward your chest while keeping your core engaged.
4. Hold the knee lift for 1-2 seconds, then lower your leg back down gently.
5. Switch to the left knee and lift it toward your chest using the same steady movement.
6. Alternate between both knees, repeating about 8-10 lifts on each side.

Wrist And Finger Movements

Wrist Rolls

- Relieves stiffness
- Increases circulation
- Enhances Flexibility and range of motion

Instructions for Wrist Rolls:

1. Sit comfortably in your chair with your feet flat on the floor and your back straight.
2. Lift your arms in front of you at chest level and extend your hands outward, palms facing down.
3. Begin by slowly rotating your wrists in a clockwise direction, making sure to move only your wrists and keeping your arms still.
4. Continue the rotations for about 10-15 seconds, then switch and rotate your wrists counterclockwise for another 10-15 seconds.
5. Keep your movements smooth and controlled to maximize the stretch without causing any discomfort.

Palm Presses

- Strengthens the Wrists and Hands
- Reduces Stiffness
- Improves Flexibility

Instructions for Palm Presses:

1. Sit comfortably in your chair with your feet flat on the floor and your back straight.
2. Bring your palms together in front of your chest in a prayer position, fingers pointing upward.

3. Press your palms firmly together while keeping your elbows up and parallel to the floor. You should feel a nice stretch in your wrists and forearms.
4. Hold the press for about 10-15 seconds, then gently release.
5. Repeat this pressing and releasing action a few times, gradually increasing the duration of the press as you become more comfortable.

Wrist Flexion and Extension

- Prevents stiffness
- Increases range of motion
- Strengthens muscles

Instructions for Wrist Flexion and Extension:

1. Sit comfortably in your chair with your feet flat on the floor and your back straight.
2. Extend your arms straight out in front of you, keeping them at shoulder height.
3. Start with your palms facing down. Slowly bend your wrists downward, pointing your fingers toward the floor. Hold this position for a few seconds to stretch the top of your wrists.
4. Then, gently bring your wrists back to the neutral position and bend them upward, pointing your fingers toward the ceiling to stretch the underside of your wrists.
5. Hold this upward position for a few seconds, then return to the neutral position.
6. Repeat this flexion and extension cycle 8-10 times, moving smoothly and at a controlled pace.

Spinal Movements

Seated Side Twist

- Releases tension in the spine
- Stimulates digestion
- Improves circulation

Instructions for Seated Side Twist:

1. Sit comfortably in your chair, ensuring that your feet are flat on the floor and your spine is erect.

2. Place your right hand on the back of the chair. Inhale, and as you exhale, gently twist your torso to the right, using your hand as leverage to deepen the twist without straining.
3. Keep your left hand on your left knee to maintain balance, and ensure your hips remain facing forward to keep the twist in the upper spine.
4. Hold the position for a few breaths, deepening the twist slightly with each exhale, but ensure you do not push beyond your comfort zone.
5. Inhale as you gently return to the center and then repeat the twist on the left side using the same method.

Side Bend

- Enhances flexibility
- Improves breathing
- Reduces spinal compression

Instructions for Side Bend:

1. Sit up straight in your chair with your feet flat on the floor, spaced comfortably apart. Ensure your hips and shoulders are aligned.
2. Extend your arms out to the sides at shoulder height.
3. Inhale deeply, and as you exhale, gently reach your right arm up and over your head, bending your torso to the left. Keep your left arm down and slightly away from your body to maintain balance.
4. Hold the position for a few seconds, feeling the stretch along your right side from your hip to your fingertips.
5. Inhale as you slowly come back up to the starting position.
6. Repeat the bend on the left side, lifting your left arm and bending toward your right.

Now that your body is warmed up and ready, let's transition into the promised chair yoga exercises, starting with exploring balance and stability poses to further enhance your strength and coordination in chair yoga.

CHAPTER 5

BALANCE AND STABILITY POSES

"Flexibility is youth."

— Diamond Dallas Page

CHAIR-ASSISTED TREE POSE

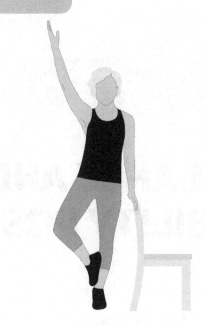

INSTRUCTIONS

1. Stand next to the chair either on the right or left of you, depending on which hand you'll use for support.
2. Using the back or seat of the chair for stability, depending on its height and your comfort level, gradually shift your weight onto the leg closest to the chair. Ensure that your feet are planted firmly on the floor. Engage your thigh and calf muscles for added stability.
3. Lift your opposite foot and rest the sole against the inner thigh or calf of your standing leg, avoiding the knee area. Keep your pelvis neutral and ensure your standing leg is strong.
4. Hold the pose, taking deep, calming breaths. Focus your gaze on a fixed point to help maintain your balance.
5. Slowly lower your raised foot back to the ground, take a deep breath, and then repeat the process on the other side.

BENEFITS

Energizes the body, strengthens the core, and provides a gentle stretch for your shoulders and back.

CHAIR PLANK POSE (PHALAKASANA)

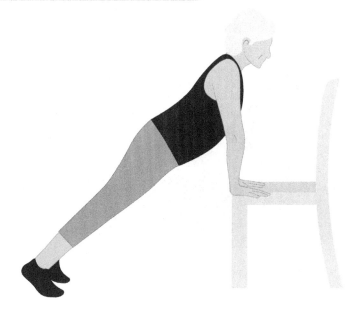

INSTRUCTIONS

1. Stand facing the chair.
2. Lean forward slightly and place your hands on the seat of the chair, positioned shoulder-width apart.
3. Slowly walk your feet back, stepping away from the chair until your body forms a straight line from head to heels.
4. Press firmly into the chair with your hands to engage your shoulders and lengthen the back of your neck.
5. Hold this position for several deep breaths, maintaining a strong and steady posture.
6. To release, walk your feet back toward the chair until you're standing upright again. Take a moment to rest, then repeat.

BENEFITS

Strengthens and tones your body, improves posture and spinal alignment, increases focus and concentration, reduces the risk of back pain, and boosts metabolism.

CHAIR BOAT POSE

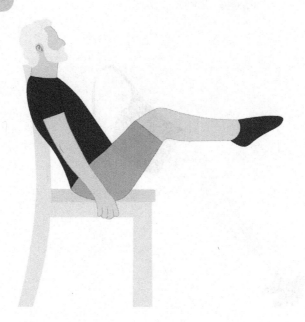

INSTRUCTIONS

1. Sit on the edge of a chair.
2. Inhale deeply, engage your core and lift your legs while leaning back slightly.
3. Grasp the sides of the chair for support.
4. Keep your abdominals firm and your spine extended.
5. Hold this position for 5-10 slow, deep breaths.

BENEFITS

Strengthens the hip flexors, abdominals, and lower spine, focuses the mind, improves overall core strength, enhances quadriceps strength, improves coordination and balance, stimulates the abdominal organs, and promotes better digestion, as well as kidney, thyroid, and prostate health.

CHAIR DOWN DOG STANDING

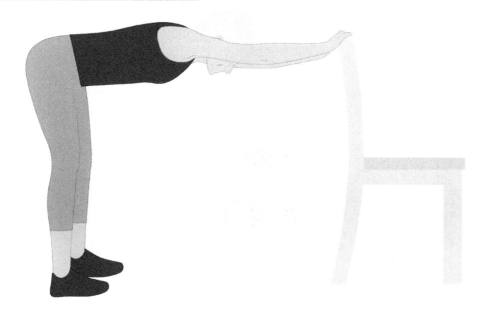

INSTRUCTIONS

1. Place a chair that can support your weight without sliding in front of you.
2. Stand facing the chair about an arm's length away, with your feet hip-width apart.
3. Place your hands on the seat of the chair.
4. As you exhale, walk your feet back until your body forms an inverted "V" shape. Keep your arms extended and parallel to the floor, with your head between your arms and looking down. Keep your neck aligned with your spine.
5. Push your hips back while pulling your chest toward the ground.
6. Hold this position, taking deep, steady breaths. Focus on lengthening your spine and feeling the stretch in your shoulders, back, and hamstrings. Stay in this position for 15-30 seconds or as long as comfortable.
7. To come out of the pose, walk your feet forward toward the chair and slowly rise to a standing position. Rest and repeat as desired.

BENEFITS

Stretches the lower body, strengthens the upper body, stimulates blood flow, and improves posture.

SEATED PALM TREE POSE WITH SIDE BEND

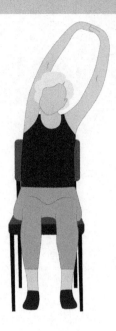

INSTRUCTIONS

1. Sit on a chair with a straight back, feet flat on the floor, and hands on your thighs.
2. Inhale deeply and slowly raise both arms overhead, keeping them straight. Either interlock your fingers or press your palms together with fingers pointing upward.
3. Exhale and gently bend your torso and arms to one side, ensuring you remain on the chair with your hips square and grounded.
4. Hold the side bend for a few breaths, feeling the stretch along the opposite side of your body.
5. Inhale and return to the center, then switch sides and repeat the bend on the other side.

BENEFITS

Improves balance and stability, enhances postural awareness, and reduces physical and mental tension.

CHAIR WARRIOR III

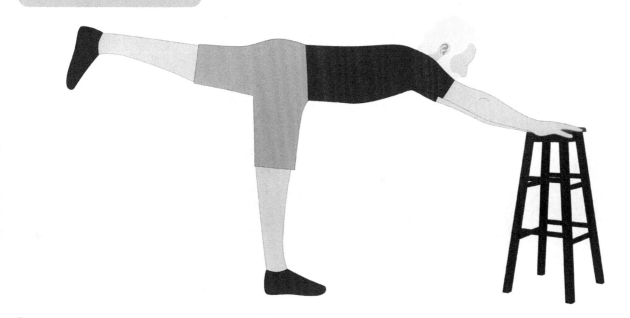

INSTRUCTIONS

1. Stand behind the chair with feet hip-width apart and hands on the back of the chair.
2. Engage your core and lift one leg straight back as you hinge forward from your hips. Aim to keep the lifted leg, torso, and head aligned and parallel to the floor.
3. As you lean forward, transfer your weight onto the standing leg, keeping a slight bend in the knee to avoid locking it.
4. Keep your hands on the chair for stability. As you grow more comfortable, extend one arm forward, parallel to the floor.
5. Maintain the pose for several breaths, focusing on steady breathing and maintaining your balance. Look down to help with stability.
6. Gently come back to the standing position and repeat on the other side.

BENEFITS

Improves balance and stability, enhances core and leg strength, and increases focus.

CHAIR FLEXING FOOT POSE

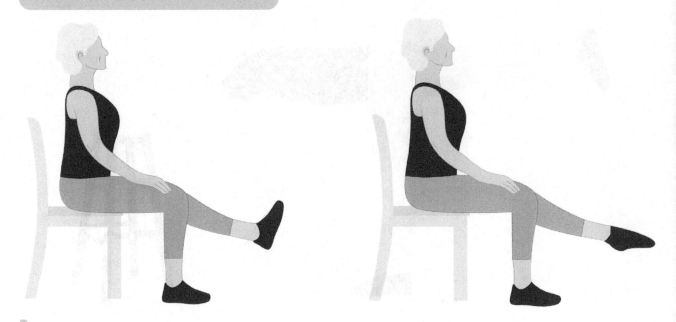

INSTRUCTIONS

1. Sit comfortably on the chair, keeping your feet flat on the floor and hip-width apart.
2. To support yourself, put your hands over your left thigh or hold the chair's side tightly.
3. Extend one leg out in front of you with your toes pointed up.
4. Push your toes back to your shin to engage your leg muscles and stretch your calf.
5. Exhale while retaining a straight back and slowly point your toes forward.
6. Maintain this posture and go through this movement 10-15 times.
7. To release, gradually sit back up while placing your right back on the floor.
8. Do this 3 times per leg, alternating each time.

BENEFITS

- Stretches muscles of leg, knee, and lower back.
- Enhance your leg's mobility and flexibility.
- Improves your stability and balance.
- Ease stiffness and tension in your lower body.
- Promotes relaxation and mindful breathing

ANKLE CRANK ON CHAIR

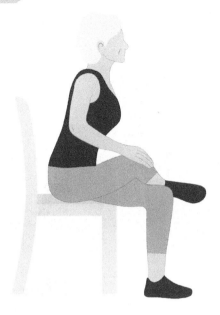

INSTRUCTIONS

1. Sit comfortably on the edge of your chair with your feet flat on the floor, hip-width apart.
2. Raise your right leg and put your right ankle over your left thigh.
3. Use your right hand to grasp your right ankle and your left hand to hold your right toes.
4. Move your right foot gently in a circular manner, starting from the ankle joint.
5. Carry out controlled and gradual rotations in one direction for about 10-15 seconds.
6. Switch directions for another 10-15 seconds.
7. Concentrate on developing smooth, full rotations to expand the stretch and movement in your ankle.
8. Slowly place your foot back on the floor and repeat on the other side.
9. Do this 3 times per leg, alternating each time.

BENEFITS

- Enhances mobility and flexibility in your ankle joint
- Boosts circulation in the feet and your lower legs
- Improves rigidness and tension in the ankles
- Helps to avoid any ankle injuries and boosts balance
- Enhances mindful mobility and relaxation

SEATED LOW LUNGE VARIATION

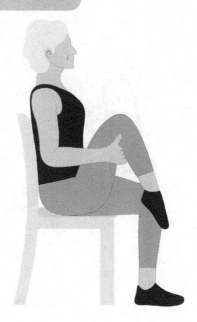

INSTRUCTIONS

1. Sit comfortably on the chair, keeping your feet flat on the floor and hip-width apart.
2. Move your left knee to your chest and grip your thigh with your hands, just under your knee.
3. Make sure that your shoulders are relaxed while keeping your back straight.
4. Take a deep breath in, lengthen your spine, and push your left knee close to your chest while exhaling to increase the stretch.
5. Maintain this position for a few deep breaths, feeling the tension loosen in your thighs and hip flexors.
6. Gradually lower your left leg to return to the starting point.
7. Repeat 3 times on each leg, alternating between the legs.

BENEFITS

- Stretches and extends thighs and hip flexors
- Boots movement flexibility in your hips
- Boosts stability and balance
- Improves tension and rigidness in hips and lower back
- Enhances mindful breathing and relaxation

INTENSE SIDE STRETCH WITH HANDS-ON CHAIR

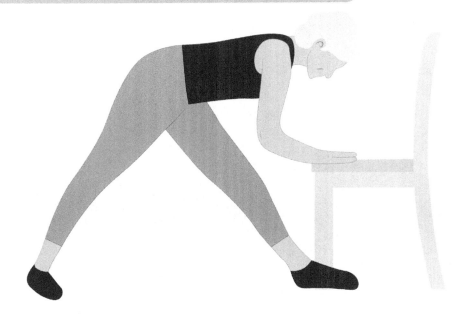

INSTRUCTIONS

1. Stand up in front of the chair.
2. Move your right foot slightly underneath the chair
3. Step your left foot back as much as you feel comfortable.
4. Move ahead slowly and put your hands on the chair seat while ensuring your arms are straight and your torso stretched.
5. Push your hands into the chair while flexing your core. Move back your left foot back more to increase the stretch.
6. Maintain this posture for a few deep breaths, keeping your body stable and aligned.
7. To release, step your back foot forward and stand up.
8. Repeat the stretch on the other side, moving your right foot back.
9. Reapest 3 times each leg, alternating each time.

BENEFITS

- Helps with strengthening and stretching the side of the body and thighs
- Enhances stability and balance
- Improves your spine and hips' flexibility
- Helps with better alignment and posture
- Boosts your energy levels and circulation

CHAPTER 6

CHAIR YOGA POSES FOR IM-PROVED MOBILITY

"In truth, yoga doesn't take time – it gives time."

– Ganga White

SEATED EAGLE POSE

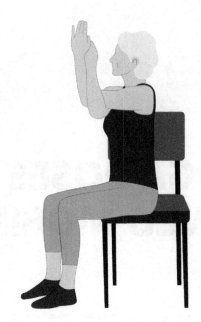

INSTRUCTIONS

1. Sit at the edge of a chair with your feet flat on the ground and your spine straight.
2. Bring your hands together in front of you with your elbows close to each other.
3. Wrap your right arm around your left arm, bringing your right palm to touch your left palm if possible.
4. Keep your spine straight and relax your shoulders.
5. Look straight ahead and breathe normally in this final position.
6. Hold the pose for as long as you are comfortable.
7. Rest and then repeat on the other side.

BENEFITS

Stretches the joints of the wrists, elbows, and shoulders, improves upper body posture, relieves stress from the shoulders and lower neck, opens up the shoulders and chest, and enhances balance.

BRIDGE POSE

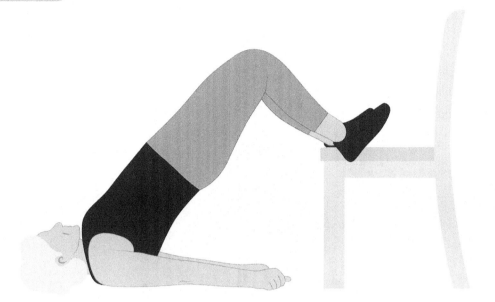

INSTRUCTIONS

1. Lie on your back on a yoga mat or other comfortable surface. Bend your knees and rest your lower legs on the seat of a chair with your knees and feet hip-width apart. Ensure that your thighs and torso form a straight line from knees to shoulders.
2. Place your arms flat on the floor alongside your body with palms facing down.
3. Press your arms and feet into the ground and lift your hips toward the ceiling.
4. Engage your core and buttocks to lift higher, but keep the movement gentle to avoid overstraining. Ensure your back stays comfortably aligned, and your neck remains relaxed.
5. Hold the lifted position for a few breaths, focusing on a smooth and steady breath.
6. Gently lower your hips back to the floor to exit the pose.

BENEFITS

Reduces back strain, increases flexibility, strength, and hip mobility, and improves blood flow.

CHAIR WARRIOR POSE 1

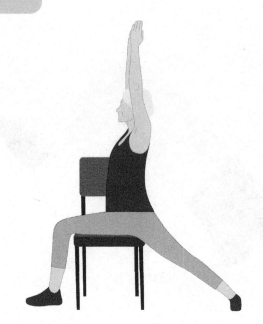

INSTRUCTIONS

1. Sit sideways on the front edge of a stable chair with one hip and leg off the chair. Reach the leg that's off the chair behind you. Plant your foot on the ground with your toes pointing outward.
2. Bend the other leg at the knee with the foot flat on the floor under the knee.
3. Adjust your hips to face forward toward your bent knee.
4. Lift your arms overhead, either parallel or with palms touching in a prayer position.
5. Engage your core to support your upper body and maintain balance.
6. Look straight ahead or slightly upward, keeping your neck long and shoulders relaxed.
7. Hold the pose for several breaths, focusing on stability and the stretch in your back, leg and hips.
8. Repeat the pose on the opposite side to ensure balance.

BENEFITS

Builds strength, improves balance and posture, provides a good stretch, and boosts energy.

HALF LOTUS POSE

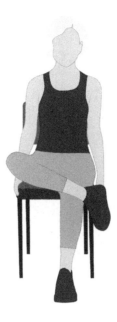

INSTRUCTIONS

1. Sit comfortably with your feet on the floor, hip-width apart.
2. Rest your hands on your thighs or knees to help maintain balance and stability.
3. Relax your shoulders away from your ears and open your chest slightly.
4. Using your hands, lift your right calf, ankle, and foot, and place them on top of your bent left leg.
5. Cushion your right foot on top of your left thigh and calf.
6. Sit up and lift your heart toward the ceiling.
7. Engage your core muscles for support.
8. Find a focal point to help you balance to maintain holding the Half Lotus position.
9. Repeat this with the opposite leg on top.

BENEFITS

Grounds and centers your energy, opens your hips, strengthens your spine and core, stretches your glutes and pelvic muscles, and promotes good posture.

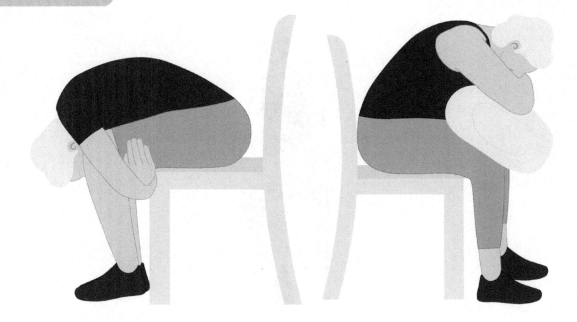

INSTRUCTIONS

1. Sit in a chair with your feet flat on the floor.
2. Inhale deeply, and as you exhale, slowly lean your torso forward from your hips, keeping your back straight.
3. Continue to lean forward, allowing your hands to rest on your knees or slide toward your ankles as you lower your torso between your legs. Your belly should rest comfortably on your thighs.
4. Let your head hang freely, releasing any tension in your neck and shoulders. Close your eyes and focus on taking deep, soothing breaths. Hold this position for several breaths or as long as it feels comfortable.

BENEFITS

Releases tension in the lower back, shoulders, and neck, lengthens and stretches the spine, and calms the central nervous system.

CHAIR MOUNTAIN POSE

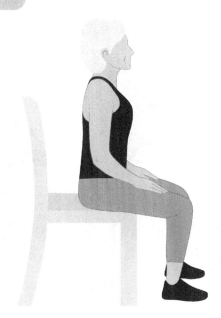

INSTRUCTIONS

1. Sit in a sturdy chair with your feet flat on the floor, hip-width apart. Straighten your back and rest your hands on your thighs.
2. Sit up, engage your core, and lengthen your spine.
3. Inhale deeply and raise your arms overhead. Either keep them parallel or bring your palms together in a prayer position.
4. Reach through your fingertips, feeling a gentle stretch in your shoulders and sides.
5. Keep your shoulders relaxed and away from your ears.
6. Hold this pose for several deep breaths, focusing on maintaining your posture and balance.
7. Exhale and slowly lower your arms back to your thighs.

BENEFITS

Improves posture, strengthens the spine and core, and enhances balance and focus.

RAGDOLL POSE

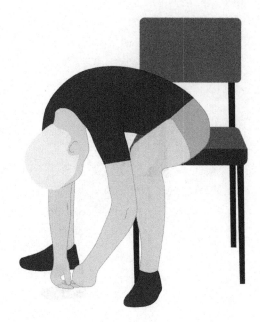

INSTRUCTIONS

1. Stand behind a sturdy chair with your feet hip-width apart.
2. Inhale deeply, and as you exhale, slowly bend forward from your hips, allowing your torso to hang down towards the floor.
3. Let your head hang freely, releasing any tension in your neck and shoulders. Hang your arms down or hold onto opposite elbows to deepen the stretch.
4. Slightly bend your knees to relieve pressure on your lower back and to make the stretch more comfortable.
5. Close your eyes if you feel steady and take several deep, relaxing breaths, feeling the gentle stretch along your spine and the back of your legs.
6. To come out of the pose, slowly roll up to a standing position, stacking each vertebra one at a time, with your head coming up last.

BENEFITS

Releases tension in the spine, neck, and shoulders, improves flexibility, and promotes relaxation.

HALF MOON POSE

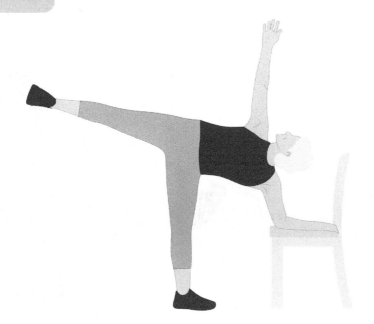

INSTRUCTIONS

1. Begin in Triangle Pose, with your right hand on your hip and your gaze down at your left foot.
2. Place your left hand on the floor in front of your left foot, or use a yoga block if reaching the floor is challenging.
3. Slowly lift your right leg until it is parallel to the floor, keeping it straight and strong.
4. Extend your right hand toward the ceiling, opening your chest and hips to the side.
5. Turn your gaze upward toward your right hand or keep your gaze forward if that helps you maintain balance.
6. Focus on lifting through the crown of your head and keep your breath steady and even.
7. Hold the pose for several breaths, then gently lower your right leg and repeat on the other side.

BENEFITS

Strengthens the core, thighs, and ankles, enhances coordination and balance, stretches the chest and shoulders for improved flexibility, and prepares the body for more challenging balancing poses.

STANDING TABLE TOP POSE WITH KNEE NOSE FLOW

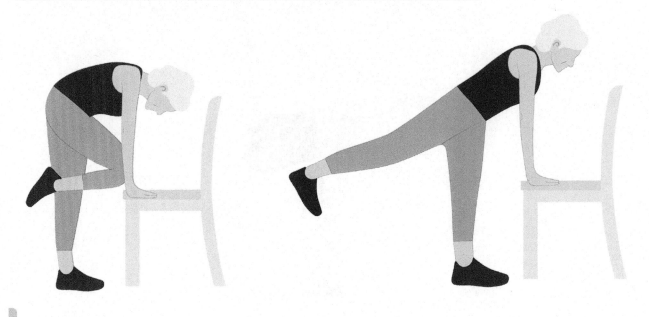

INSTRUCTIONS

1. Stand up in front of your chair.
2. Put your hands on the seat, shoulder-width apart.
3. Stretch your feet back until your body is straight, forming a modified plank posture from head to heels.
4. While inhaling, raise your right leg straight back, maintaining your hips level.
5. While exhaling, bring your left knee to your chest, circulating your back slowly..
6. While inhaling, extend your right leg back again, getting back to the straight-line posture.
7. Repeat this action for a few deep breaths, then repeat on the other leg.
8. Repeat 3-5 times per leg, alternating each time.

BENEFITS

- Builds your core muscles and enhances stability
- Improves coordination and balance
- Stretches and strengthens the thighs and hip muscles
- Increase hips and lower back flexibility
- Promotes breath awareness and mindful movement

SEATED EXTENDED SIDE ANGLE

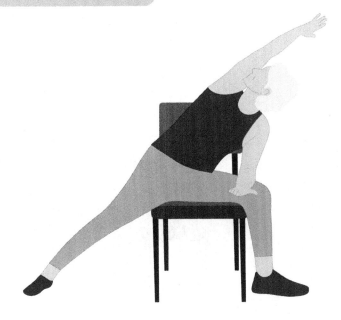

INSTRUCTIONS

1. Sit on your chair comfortably while placing your feet flat on the floor.
2. Extend your right leg out to the side, keeping your foot flat on the floor. Bend your left knee at a 90-degree angle, keeping your left foot flat on the floor.
3. Put your left forearm over your left thigh, ensuring your shoulder is relaxed.
4. Stretch your right arm toward the ceiling, then gradually bend to your left, stretching your right arm over your head and extending it towards your right side.
5. Maintain this stretch for a few deep breaths, feeling the stretch all along your right side.
6. To release, bring your right arm and right leg back to the starting position.
7. Repeat the stretch on the other side by stretching your left leg outward and stretching with your left arm.
8. Repeat 3-5 times each side, alternating each time.

BENEFITS

- Stretches the torso's side and hips
- Boosts flexibility and movement in the spine
- Improves overall stability and balance
- Enhances body alignment and posture
- Promotes deep and mindful breathing

GODDESS POSE CHAIR SIDE STRETCH

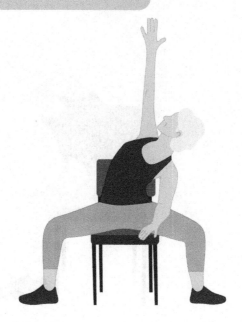

INSTRUCTIONS

1. Sit on your chair comfortably while placing your feet flat on the floor.
2. Point your knees out at a 90-degree angle, keeping your feet flat on the floor, placing your hands on your thighs.
3. Bend to your right side, moving your right hand down towards your right thigh in the direction of your knee and breathing deeply throughout.
4. Lift your left arm upon your head, extending towards the right side. Ultimately, feel the stretch along your left side.
5. Maintain this posture for a few deep breaths, holding a straight spine and engaging your core.
6. Repeat the same movement reversed on your other side. Do this 3-5 times per side, alternating each time.

BENEFITS

- Stretches and opens the inner thighs, hips, and groin
- Improved spine flexibility and torso mobility
- Strengthen the core and legs' muscles
- Enhances body alignment and posture
- Improves conscious and deep breathing

CHAPTER 7

CHAIR YOGA POSES FOR STRENGTH BUILDING

"Most people have no idea how good their body is designed to feel."

— Kevin Trudeau

SINGLE LEG FORWARD BEND (CHAIR JANU SIRSASANA)

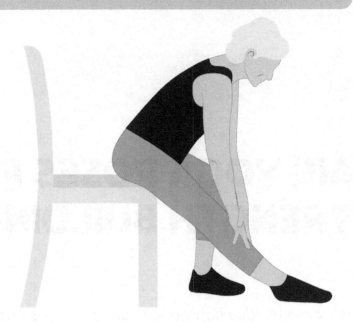

INSTRUCTIONS

1. Sit comfortably on a sturdy chair with your feet flat on the ground and your spine straight.
2. Extend one leg straight in front of you. Either rest it on the ground or another chair. Keep the other foot flat on the ground for stability. Make sure the extended leg is straight but not locked at the knee. A slight bend can help maintain good posture.
3. Engage your abdominal muscles to support your spine. This will help you maintain balance and protect your back as you bend forward.
4. Inhale and lengthen your spine. On the exhale, gently hinge forward from your hips over the extended leg. Extend your arms toward your foot as far as comfortable, making sure not to round your back.
5. Hold this position and take deep, steady breaths. Feel the stretch in your lower back and the gentle pull in your extended leg.
6. Inhale to come back up to an upright position, then exhale and bring your arms down to your sides.
7. Repeat the pose with the other leg extended.

BENEFITS

Stretches the lower back, massages the abdominal organs, and tones the shoulders.

GLUTE STRETCH (CHAIR PIGEON POSE)

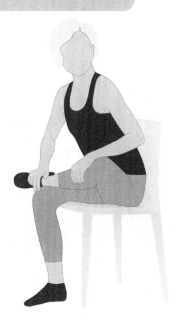

INSTRUCTIONS

1. Sit up in a sturdy chair. Ensure your back is straight, shoulders relaxed, and feet flat on the floor to set a stable base.
2. Lift your right ankle and rest it on your left thigh, just above the knee. Ensure your right knee is aligned with your right ankle to prevent any strain.
3. Keep your spine straight as you gently press your right knee down with your hand to deepen the stretch in your right hip. This helps open up the hip area while you're supported by the chair.
4. Maintain this position, taking slow, deep breaths to relax into the stretch.
5. After holding the pose for a few breaths, switch sides to balance the stretch.

BENEFITS

Enhances flexibility, alleviates lower back pain, and promotes relaxation.

CHAIR YOGA LUNGE POSE

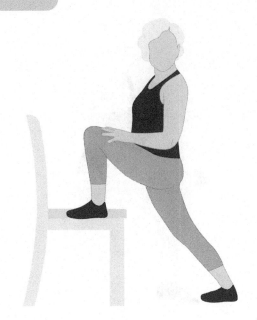

INSTRUCTIONS

1. Place a sturdy chair in front of you, facing toward you.
2. Stand facing the chair at a comfortable distance. Slowly lift one leg and place your foot fully on the seat of the chair. Ensure your hips are squared to the front and your standing leg is straight and strong.
3. Place your hands on your hips or extend them outward or upward to help with balance. Keep your spine elongated and your gaze forward.
4. Focus on evenly distributing your weight and maintaining a steady breath. Engage your core to support your upper body.
5. Carefully lower your leg back to the standing position. Repeat the pose with the opposite leg to ensure balanced exercise.

BENEFITS

Strengthens the lower body, improves flexibility and range of motion, enhances balance and stability, and supports joint health.

HALF-SPLIT POSE WITH A CHAIR

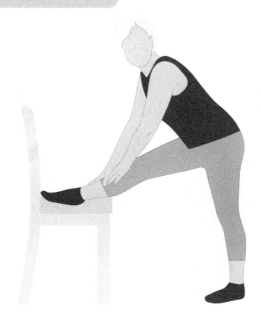

INSTRUCTIONS

1. Stand in front of a chair with enough room to comfortably extend one leg onto the seat.
2. Place one heel on the seat. The extended leg should be straight with toes flexed toward you and aligned with your hip.
3. Focus on balancing and stabilizing your standing leg.
4. Walk your hands down your extended leg and hinge forward from your hips into a gentle forward fold.
5. Hold the position for a few breaths, then bring your torso back to an upright position.
6. Repeat the pose with the opposite leg to ensure balanced stretching.

BENEFITS

Improves balance and stability, reduces pain symptoms, decreases the number of falls, and enhances mental well-being and confidence.

SEATED SHOULDER SHRUGS

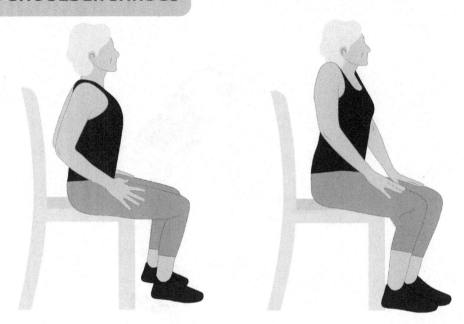

INSTRUCTIONS

1. Sit with a straight spine straight and feet flat on the floor.
2. Raise your shoulders toward your ears. Hold the position for a few seconds.
3. Slowly lower your shoulders back down to their normal position.
4. Inhale deeply as you lift your shoulders, and exhale as you release them for added relaxation.
5. Perform this movement several times in a row, taking a short rest between sets, and then repeat the exercise.

BENEFITS

Relieves shoulder tension and strengthens the shoulder and trapezius muscles.

SEATED SHOULDER PRESS

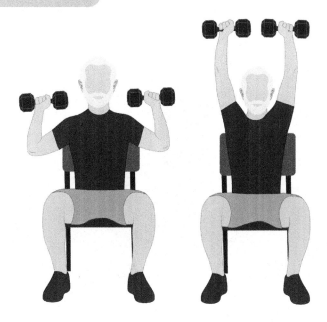

INSTRUCTIONS

1. Sit in a sturdy chair with a straight back and feet flat on the floor.
2. Hold a pair of light dumbbells or water bottles with your palms facing outward. Ensure the weight is comfortable enough to allow you to complete the exercise without discomfort. Start with your hands at shoulder level, and elbows bent and pointing out to the sides. Make sure your wrists are straight.
3. Exhale and press the weights upward until your arms are fully extended overhead. Keep your wrists straight and your back firmly against the chair. Ensure that you do this as a slow, controlled movement to avoid straining your shoulder joints.
4. Inhale as you slowly lower the weights back to the starting position at shoulder level.

BENEFITS

Improves shoulder mobility and strengthens your shoulder muscles.

SEATED CAMEL POSE

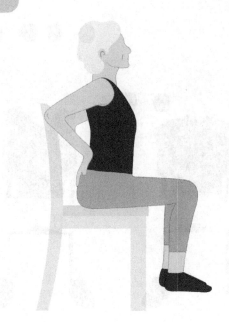

INSTRUCTIONS

1. Sit in a chair with your feet flat on the floor, spaced hip-distance apart. Keep your spine straight with your hands on your knees.
2. Extend your arms back and gently grasp the back legs of the chair.
3. Slowly push your pelvis forward and arch your back, lifting your sternum toward the ceiling to open your chest.
4. Let your head gently drop back.
5. Hold the position for a few deep breaths, allowing your backbend to deepen with each exhale.
6. Carefully bring your hands back to your knees and sit upright. Take a moment to let your body adjust.

BENEFITS

Improves spinal flexibility, opens the chest, and stretches the shoulders and front body.

DOLPHIN POSE FOREARMS ON CHAIR

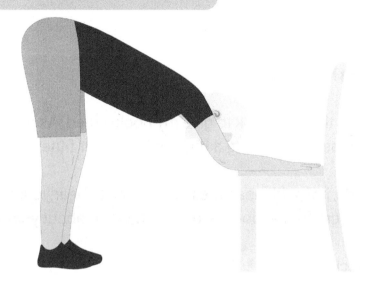

INSTRUCTIONS

1. Stand with the chair in front of you, approximately at the distance of arm's length.
2. Put your forearms on the seat while keeping your elbows shoulder-width apart.
3. Extend your legs backward until your body forms an inverted "V" shape, elevating your hips toward the ceiling.
4. Slightly bend your knees while stretching your heels toward the floor.
5. Push into your forearms while engaging your core to stretch your spine and open your shoulders.
6. Allow your head to hang freely among your arms while relaxing your neck.
7. Maintain this position for a few deep breaths, feeling a stretch in your back, thighs, and hamstrings.
8. To release, gradually move your feet backward toward the chair until you stand upright. Do the movement 3-5 times.

BENEFITS

- Opens the shoulders, thighs, legs, and arches of the feet
- Strengthen the arms, core, and shoulders
- Enhance body alignment and posture
- Eases tension in the upper body
- Improves balance and stability

Thank you for making it this far!

I greatly appreciate the time you took to give my book a read. As a small indie publisher, it means a lot and I hope I am making a difference in your fitness journey.

If you have 60 seconds, it would mean the world to me to hear your honest feedback on Amazon. It does wonders for the book and I love hearing about your experience with it!

To leave your feedback:

- Open your camera app
- Point your mobile device at the QR code below
- The review page will appear in your web browser

You can also leave your feedback under your Amazon orders page.

Thank you!

CHAPTER 8

CHAIR YOGA FOR MINDFULNESS AND RELAXATION

"Yoga is the journey of the self, through the self, to the self."

— *The Bhagavad Gita*

SEATED FORWARD BEND

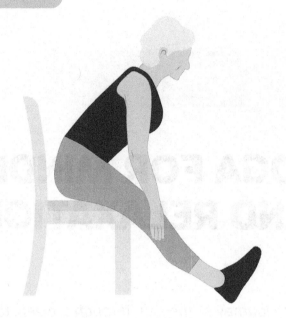

INSTRUCTIONS

1. Sit at the edge of a chair with your feet flat on the floor, spaced comfortably apart.
2. Inhale deeply and lengthen your spine.
3. Exhale and hinge forward from your hips, keeping your back straight.
4. Walk your hands forward along your legs or the floor as far as is comfortable, allowing a gentle stretch.
5. With each inhale, lift and lengthen your chest slightly. With each exhale, allow yourself to relax more into the forward bend.
6. Stay in the pose for 15-30 seconds, then gently come back up to a sitting position. Rest for a moment and repeat if desired.

BENEFITS

Stretches the spine, hamstrings, and calves, calms the mind, and stimulates internal organs.

SEATED SIDE BEND

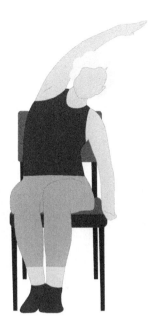

INSTRUCTIONS

1. Sit upright in a sturdy chair with your feet flat on the ground.
2. Place your left hand on the chair seat or floor beside you with your elbow slightly bent for support.
3. Reach your right arm up and over your head, leaning gently to the left side.
4. Hold this position for 30 seconds to 1 minute, focusing on deep, even breaths.
5. Return to the starting position, then repeat the stretch on the opposite side.

BENEFITS

Strengthens the spine and core muscles, stretches the side torso, targets the lymph nodes in the armpit and lymphatic organs, and releases tension in the ribs.

CHAIR CAT-COW STRETCH

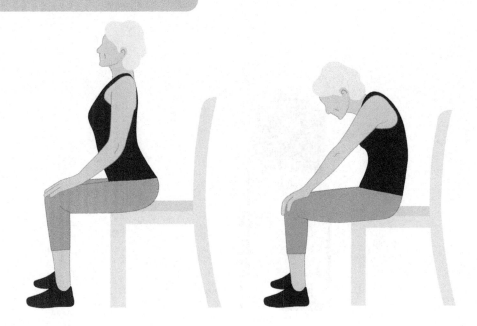

INSTRUCTIONS

1. Sit toward the front edge of a sturdy chair. Keep your feet flat on the floor and your knees aligned over your ankles.
2. Sit up straight and place your hands just above your knees.
3. Inhale as you move your hands forward on your knees, tuck your chin toward your chest, and arch your back. This is the cat pose.
4. Transition to the cow pose by exhaling as you move your hands back to the starting position, lifting your head slowly, and straightening your spine.
5. Perform this sequence slowly 3-5 times. Rest for a few minutes and repeat for a total of 3 sets.

BENEFITS

Calms the mind, relieves stress, opens the chest, and stretches the abdomen, back, spine, and upper neck.

SEATED SPINAL TWIST

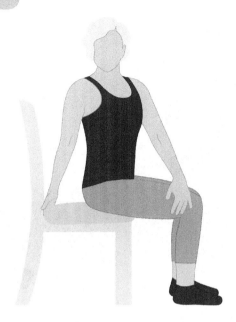

INSTRUCTIONS

1. Sit comfortably on the edge or middle of a sturdy chair with your feet flat on the floor to create a strong foundation. Keep your spine straight and your shoulders relaxed.
2. Engage your core slightly to support your lower back during the twist.
3. Place your right hand on the back of the chair for support.
4. Inhale to lengthen your spine, and as you exhale, gently twist to the right. Use your right hand for leverage to deepen the twist gradually without forcing it. Look over your right shoulder if it is comfortable to do so.
5. Hold the twist for a few breaths, maintaining a long spine and relaxed shoulders.
6. Slowly return to the center on an inhale and repeat the twist on the left side.

BENEFITS

Improves spinal mobility, aids in digestion, and helps release tension in the back and shoulders.

SEATED CORPSE POSE

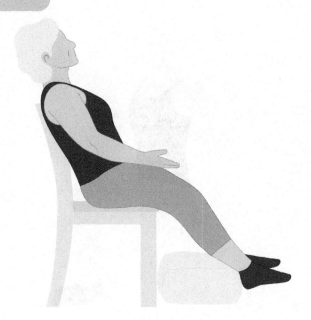

INSTRUCTIONS

1. Sit in a chair with your back supported by the backrest and your feet flat on the floor.
2. Let your arms rest on your thighs or alongside the chair with palms facing up.
3. Close your eyes and take deep, slow breaths.
4. Relax each part of your body from your face to your feet, consciously releasing tension with each exhale. Allow your body to feel heavy and fully supported by the chair.

BENEFITS

Reduces stress, calms the mind, improves mental clarity, lowers blood pressure, and promotes overall relaxation.

LEGS-ON-THE-CHAIR POSE

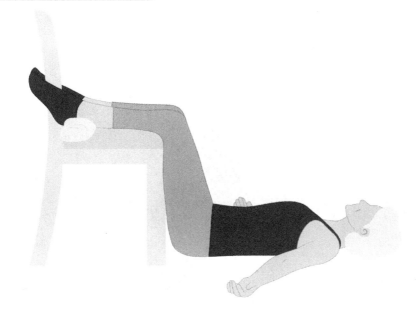

INSTRUCTIONS

1. Set up a chair near a wall or in a space where it won't slide. Place a yoga mat or blanket on the floor in front of the chair for cushioning.
2. Sit down on the mat with your back to the chair, close enough so that when you lie back, your legs rest comfortably on the seat.
3. Slowly lower your back onto the mat while lifting your legs to place them on the chair. Your calves should rest on the seat, creating a 90-degree angle at your knees.
4. Make sure your lower legs are supported by the chair and your knees are bent at about a 90-degree angle.
5. Let your arms rest by your sides with palms facing up, or place them on your belly.
6. Close your eyes and focus on deep, slow belly breaths. Allow your body to relax completely with each exhale.

BENEFITS

Promotes physical relaxation, improves circulation, and relieves stress.

SEATED MOUNTAIN POSE WITH OVERHEAD STRETCH

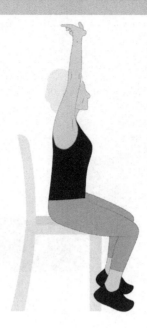

INSTRUCTIONS

1. Sit comfortably with your feet flat on the floor and your spine straight.
2. Inhale deeply and slowly raise your arms overhead, with your palms facing each other.
3. Gently stretch upward as if trying to touch the ceiling, feeling the length of your spine and sides.
4. Hold the stretch for a few seconds, then exhale and lower your arms. Rest for a moment.
5. Repeat this movement 3-5 times, focusing on your breath and the stretch.

BENEFITS

Stretches the sides and back, helps with focus and deep breathing, and promotes relaxation.

BOUND ANGLE POSE I

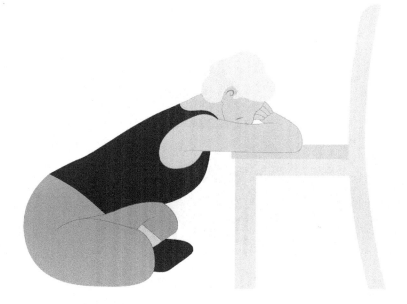

INSTRUCTIONS

1. Sit comfortably on the floor facing a chair with your legs in front of you.
2. Bring your feet soles together, allowing your knees to open to the sides like a butterfly.
3. Move a bit closer to the chair so you can easily incline forward and relax your head and forearms on the chair's seat.
4. Rest your neck and head on the chair to allow them to relax.
5. Take a deep breath and maintain this position for a few breaths until you feel the stretch in your hips and inner thighs.

BENEFITS

- Strengthen the groin and inner thighs
- Enhances hips' flexibility
- Improves relaxation and relieves stress
- Offers gentle support for neck and back
- Increase lower body's circulation

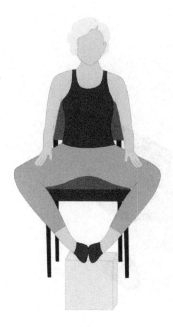

INSTRUCTIONS

1. Sit comfortably over your chair's edge while placing your feet flat on the floor.
2. Move the soles of your feet together, opening your knees to the side.
3. Sit up straight and engage your core while relaxing your shoulders.
4. Gently push your knees towards the floor to increase the stretch within your inner thighs.
5. Maintain this posture for a few deep breaths, keeping a straight back and balanced posture.
6. While releasing, bring your knees in and move your feet back to the floor.
7. Repeat the stretch 3-5 times.

BENEFITS

- Extends the groin and inner thighs
- Enhances hips' flexibility
- Improves spinal alignment and body posture
- Boosts lower body's circulation
- Facilitates in relieving stress and tension

CHAPTER 9

CHAIR YOGA ROUTINES FOR SENIORS

"First, forget inspiration. Habit is more dependable. Habit will sustain you whether you're inspired or not."

- Octavia Butler

In the previous chapter, we discussed many effective chair yoga poses for you to explore and try. Now, it's time to bring it all together in the 21-day challenge. From there, we will learn how to make our own routines.

The 21-Day Challenge

Welcome to your 21-day chair yoga challenge! Each day, we'll focus on different aspects of yoga, starting with a gentle introduction and warm-up. Let's get moving and enjoy this journey together!

You can track your progress with the 21-day challenge tracker which you can find at the end of this chapter, or you can download and print it out here:

(Scan with your phone or ipad camera)

Resting is as important as the workouts themselves. As you will notice, I didn't provide any rest days. Everyone's body heals differently and what might work for one person won't necessarily work for another. Ensure you listen to your body and rest when you need to. Anywhere from 2-4 days a week will work fine. Improving our health isn't a sprint but a marathon. Take it slow and enjoy the process!

Goodluck, be safe, and most importantly have fun!

Day 1: Gentle Introduction and Warm-Up

Warm-Up (5 minutes)

1. **Deep Breathing (3 minutes):** Sit comfortably, inhale deeply through your nose, and exhale slowly through your mouth. Feel the breath calming your mind and body.
2. **Neck Stretches (2 minutes):** Gently tilt your head toward each shoulder, forward, and back, holding each position for 5 seconds.

Main Workout (15 minutes)

1. **Seated Cat-Cow Stretch (6 minutes):** Inhale as you arch your back and look up (Cow Pose), then exhale as you round your spine and tuck your chin (Cat Pose). Repeat slowly for 2 minutes, take a 30-second rest, and repeat 3 times.
2. **Seated Side Stretch (3 minutes each side):** Extend one arm overhead and lean to the opposite side. Hold for 20 seconds and switch sides after 3 minutes.
3. **Chair Flexing Foot Pose (3 minutes each side)** Extend one leg and point your toes. Hold, then flex your toes back for a stretch. Repeat 15 times, then switch legs. Rest and repeat 3 times for each side.

Cool Down (5 minutes)

1. **Deep Breathing in Corpse Pose (3 minutes):** Continue with deep, slow breaths, focusing on relaxation.
2. **Seated Meditation (2 minutes):** Close your eyes, focus on your breath, and clear your mind.

Day 2: Focus on Upper Body Flexibility

Warm-Up (5 minutes)

1. **Shoulder Rolls (2 minutes):** Slowly roll your shoulders forward and backward 10 times in each direction to release tension and warm up your shoulder joints.
2. **Arm Lifts (3 minutes):** Raise your arms overhead slowly, hold for 2 seconds, then lower them. Repeat 15 times to stretch and strengthen your shoulders.

Main Workout (15 minutes)

1. **Seated Twist (5 minutes):** Twist your torso to one side and hold for 20 seconds, then switch sides. Repeat 8 times on each side to enhance flexibility.
2. **Seated Eagle Arms (5 minutes):** Cross your arms and press your palms together. Hold for 30 seconds, then switch arms. Repeat 4 times on each side to stretch your upper back and shoulders.
3. **Wrist and Finger Stretches (5 minutes):** Extend your fingers, then flex into a fist, holding each position for 10 seconds. Rotate your wrists 10 times in each direction to increase flexibility.

Cool Down (5 minutes)

1. **Gentle Neck Rolls (3 minutes):** Roll your head around your neck slowly 5 times in each direction to relax your neck muscles.
2. **Arm Stretches (2 minutes):** Extend one arm across your body and hold for 20 seconds, then switch arms. Repeat 3 times each arm to stretch your shoulders and upper back.

Day 3: Lower Body Strength

Warm-Up (5 minutes)

1. **Ankle Rolls (2 minutes):** Sit comfortably and rotate each ankle slowly, 10 times in each direction. This will help loosen up your ankles and prepare them for the workout.
2. **Knee Lifts (3 minutes):** Lift one knee toward your chest, hold for 2 seconds, then switch legs. Repeat 15 times for each leg. You can hold the sides of your seat for stability.

Main Workout (15 minutes)

1. **Seated Leg Lifts (5 minutes):** Extend one leg straight out, hold for 5 seconds, then lower it. Repeat 10 times for each leg. Take a brief rest and then repeat for 3 sets.
2. **Ankle Stretches (5 minutes):** Point your toes forward, hold for 5 seconds, then flex your foot back, holding for another 5 seconds. Repeat 10 times for each foot.
3. **Chair Squats (5 minutes):** Stand up and sit down on your chair carefully, focusing on controlled movements. Repeat 10 times to strengthen your legs.

Cool Down (5 minutes)

1. **Leg and Calf Stretch (3 minutes):** Extend one leg straight out and reach towards your toe. Hold for 20 seconds, then switch legs. Repeat 3 times for each leg.
2. **Deep Breathing (2 minutes):** Sit back, close your eyes, and focus on slow, deep breaths. Inhale for 5 seconds, hold and then exhale for 5 seconds.

Day 4: Core Engagement

Warm-Up (5 minutes)

1. **Side Bends (3 minutes):** Reach one arm overhead and bend to the side. Hold for 10 seconds, then switch sides. Alternate sides for 3 minutes, taking a brief rest every 30 seconds.
2. **Seated Marching (2 minutes):** Lift your knees alternately as if marching, holding each lift for 1 second. Continue for 2 minutes to engage your core.

Main Workout (15 minutes)

1. **Seated Pelvic Tilts (5 minutes):** Tilt your pelvis forward, hold for 5 seconds, then tilt it back and hold for 5 seconds. Repeat this movement 15 times to engage your lower abdominal muscles.
2. **Abdominal Bracing (5 minutes):** Tighten your abdominal muscles as if bracing for impact. Hold for 10 seconds, then relax for 5 seconds. Repeat this 20 times.
3. **Seated Side Twists (5 minutes):** Twist your torso to one side, hold for 10 seconds, then switch sides. Repeat 10 times on each side to work your oblique muscles.

Cool Down (5 minutes)

1. **Full Body Stretch (3 minutes):** Extend your arms overhead and stretch your legs out. Hold this stretch for 10 seconds, then relax. Repeat 5 times to lengthen your entire body.
2. **Deep Breathing (2 minutes):** Inhale deeply for 5 seconds and then exhale for 5 seconds. Repeat this 10 times to calm your mind and body.

Day 5: Balance and Stability

Warm-Up (5 minutes)

1. **Toe Taps (2 minutes):** Sit comfortably and tap your toes on the floor rapidly. Keep this up for 2 minutes to get your legs moving and warmed up.
2. **Heel Raises (3 minutes):** Lift your heels off the floor, hold for 3 seconds, and then lower them. Repeat this 20 times to warm up your calves and ankles.

Main Workout (15 minutes)

1. **Single-Leg Lifts (5 minutes):** Extend one leg out straight, hold for 5 seconds, then switch to the other leg. Repeat 10 times for each leg.
2. **Chair Plank Pose (5 minutes):** Place your hands on the chair arms or seat and hold your body in a plank position for 10 seconds. Then walk your feet forward to stand up. Rest for 30 seconds and repeat this sequence 5 times.
3. **Warrior Pose I (5 minutes):** Extend one leg to the side and stretch your arms out. Hold this pose for 20 seconds, then switch sides. Repeat 3 times for each side.

Cool Down (5 minutes)

1. **Seated Forward Bend (3 minutes):** Lean forward from your hips and reach toward the floor. Hold this stretch for 20 seconds and repeat 3 times.
2. **Deep Breathing (2 minutes):** Sit comfortably, inhale deeply for 5 seconds, and exhale for 5 seconds. Repeat this 10 times to relax.

Day 6: Gentle Flow

Warm-Up (5 minutes)

1. **Neck Tilts (2 minutes):** Gently tilt your head toward each shoulder, holding for 5 seconds on each side. Repeat this 5 times per side to release neck tension.
2. **Shoulder Shrugs (3 minutes):** Lift your shoulders toward your ears, hold for 3 seconds, and then release. Repeat 20 times to loosen up your shoulders.

Main Workout (15 minutes)

1. **Flow Between Seated Cat-Cow (7 minutes):** Alternate between arching your back (Cow Pose) and rounding your spine (Cat Pose). Hold each position for 5 seconds and continue flowing smoothly for 7 minutes.
2. **Seated Mountain to Forward Bend (8 minutes):** Sit and stretch your arms overhead (Mountain Pose), hold for 5 seconds, then lean forward into a forward bend, holding for another 5 seconds. Repeat this 10 times to enhance flexibility and relaxation.
3. **Seated Twists (3 minutes)** Twist your torso to one side, using the chair's seat or backrest for support. Hold for a few breaths, then switch sides. Repeat for 3 minutes, resting when needed.

Cool Down (5 minutes)

1. **Wrist and Finger Stretches (3 minutes):** Extend and flex your wrists, then curl and stretch your fingers. Hold each position for 5 seconds and repeat 10 times to stretch your hands and wrists.
2. **Seated Meditation (2 minutes):** Close your eyes, focus on your breath, and clear your mind. Sit still and enjoy this peaceful moment.

Day 7: Mindfulness and Breathwork

Warm-Up (5 minutes)

1. **Gentle Neck Rolls (3 minutes):** Sit comfortably and gently roll your head around your neck, 5 times in each direction. This will help release any tension.
2. **Shoulder Shrugs (2 minutes):** Lift your shoulders toward your ears, hold for 3 seconds, then release. Repeat this 15 times to warm up your shoulders.

Main Workout (15 minutes)

1. **Guided Breathing Exercises (7 minutes):** Focus on your breath. Inhale deeply for 5 seconds, hold for 3 seconds, then exhale slowly for 7 seconds. Continue this pattern for 7 minutes to calm your mind and body.
2. **Seated Twist and Gentle Side Stretches (8 minutes):** Twist gently to each side, holding each twist for 10 seconds. Follow this with a gentle side stretch, holding for 10 seconds on each side. Repeat this sequence 8 times for each side to enhance flexibility and mindfulness.
3. **Half-wind Release Pose (3 minutes)** Lift one knee towards your chest, holding it with your hands for support. Hold for a few breaths, then switch legs. Do this for 3 minutes, resting when necessary.

Cool Down (5 minutes)

1. **Guided Relaxation (3 minutes):** Sit comfortably, listen to soothing music, or follow a guided imagery session to relax fully.
2. **Meditation (2 minutes):** Close your eyes, focus on calming thoughts, and breathe naturally. Let your mind relax and enjoy the peace.

Day 8: Upper Body Strength

Warm-Up (5 minutes)

1. **Arm Circles (3 minutes):** Extend your arms to the sides and make small circles, gradually making them larger. Do this for 1 minute in each direction to warm up your shoulders.

2. **Shoulder Stretches (2 minutes):** Bring one arm across your body and hold it with the other hand, stretching for 10 seconds on each side. Repeat this stretch 3 times for each side to loosen up your shoulders.

Main Workout (15 minutes)

1. **Seated Rowing (5 minutes):** Pretend you're rowing a boat with your arms. Squeeze your shoulder blades together with each 'row' and hold for 3 seconds. Repeat this 20 times to strengthen your upper back.
2. **Arm Raises (5 minutes):** Lift your arms to shoulder height and then overhead. Hold each position for 2 seconds before lowering them. Repeat this 15 times to build shoulder strength. Rest, then do 2 more sets of 15.
3. **Tricep Stretches (5 minutes):** Reach one hand down your back and gently push your elbow with the other hand. Hold this stretch for 20 seconds on each side and repeat 3 times to stretch your triceps.

Cool Down (5 minutes)

1. **Neck Stretches (3 minutes):** Tilt your head toward each shoulder and hold for 10 seconds on each side. Repeat this 3 times per side to release neck tension.
2. **Deep Breathing (2 minutes):** Sit comfortably and focus on your breath. Inhale deeply for 5 seconds, then exhale for 5 seconds. Repeat this 10 times to end your session feeling relaxed and refreshed.

Day 9: Leg Flexibility

Warm-Up (5 minutes)

1. **Knee Hugs (3 minutes):** Sit comfortably and pull one knee at a time toward your chest, holding for 5 seconds. Alternate sides and repeat 10 times per leg to warm up your hips and lower back.
2. **Leg Swings (2 minutes):** Stand behind your chair and gently swing each leg back and forth, holding onto the chair for balance. Do 10 swings per leg to loosen up your legs.

Main Workout (15 minutes)

1. **Seated Hamstring Stretch (5 minutes):** Extend one leg out in front of you, then slowly lean forward from your hips. Hold the stretch for 20 seconds and repeat 3 times for each leg to stretch your hamstrings.
2. **Chair Flexing Foot Pose (5 minutes):** Extend one leg, pushing the heel away and pulling the toes toward you. Hold for 20 seconds then push the toes away from you. Repeat 3 times per leg to stretch your calves.
3. **Seated Pigeon Pose (5 minutes):** Place one ankle over the opposite knee and lean forward gently. Hold for 20 seconds and repeat 3 times on each side to open your hips.

Cool Down (5 minutes)

1. **Ankle Rolls (3 minutes):** Rotate your ankles in both directions, 10 times each. Switch your legs and repeat to relax your ankles.
2. **Deep Breathing (2 minutes):** Sit comfortably and focus on your breath. Inhale for 5 seconds and exhale for 5 seconds. Repeat this 10 times to end your session feeling relaxed.

Day 10: Spinal Health

Warm-Up (5 minutes)

1. **Seated Twists (3 minutes):** Sit up and gently twist to each side, holding for 2-3 seconds. Alternate sides and repeat 6 times per side to warm up your spine.
2. **Side Bends (2 minutes):** Reach one arm overhead and bend to the side, holding for 10 seconds. Repeat 3 times per side to stretch your sides.

Main Workout (15 minutes)

1. **Seated Cat-Cow Stretch (6 minutes):** Sit comfortably and arch your back while looking up (Cow Pose), then round your spine and tuck your chin (Cat Pose). Hold each position for 5 seconds and repeat 15 times to improve spinal flexibility.

2. **Gentle Backbends (5 minutes):** Inhale and lean back slightly, holding the position for 10 seconds. Return to the starting position and repeat 10 times to strengthen your back.
3. **Spinal Twist (4 minutes):** Sit up and twist gently to each side, holding for 10 seconds. Repeat 8 times per side to enhance spinal mobility.

Cool Down (5 minutes)

1. **Full Back Stretch (3 minutes):** Extend your arms and legs, lean forward, and hold for 15 seconds. Repeat 3 times to stretch your entire back.
2. **Deep Breathing (2 minutes):** Sit comfortably and focus on slow, deep breaths. Inhale and exhale for 10 cycles to finish your session feeling calm and relaxed.

Day 11: Enhanced Flexibility

Warm-Up (5 minutes)

1. **Arm and Leg Reaches (3 minutes):** Sit comfortably and extend your opposite arm and leg, holding the stretch for 5 seconds. Alternate sides and repeat 10 times each to warm up your limbs.
2. **Seated Twists (2 minutes):** Twist your upper body to each side, holding for 10 seconds. Repeat 5 times per side to loosen up your spine.

Main Workout (15 minutes)

1. **Seated Forward Bend (5 minutes):** Lean forward from your hips and reach toward your toes, holding for 20 seconds. Repeat 5 times to stretch your hamstrings and lower back.
2. **Seated Side Stretch (5 minutes):** Extend one arm overhead and lean to the side, holding for 15 seconds. Alternate sides and repeat 4 times each to stretch your sides.
3. **Neck and Shoulder Stretches (5 minutes):** Gently tilt your head toward each shoulder and hold for 10 seconds. Then, roll your shoulders slowly, repeating 10 times to release tension.

Cool Down (5 minutes)

1. **Full Body Relaxation (3 minutes):** Close your eyes and relax each body part sequentially from head to toe.

2. **Deep Breathing (2 minutes):** Sit comfortably and focus on your breath. Inhale deeply for 5 seconds and exhale for 5 seconds, repeating 10 times to finish your session feeling calm.

Day 12: Core and Back Strengthening

Warm-Up (5 minutes)

1. **Pelvic Tilts (3 minutes):** Sit comfortably and tilt your pelvis forward and back, holding each tilt for 5 seconds. Repeat 15 times to warm up your lower back.
2. **Seated Marching (2 minutes):** Lift your knees alternately as if marching, holding each lift for 1 second. Continue for 2 minutes to engage your core.

Main Workout (15 minutes)

1. **Abdominal Twists (5 minutes):** Twist your torso to each side, holding for 10 seconds. Repeat 10 times per side to strengthen your core.
2. **Boat Pose (5 minutes):** From a seated position, lean back slightly and hold the pose for 10 seconds. Repeat 10 times to engage your abdominal muscles.
3. **Pelvic Floor Exercises (5 minutes):** Tighten your pelvic floor muscles, holding for 5 seconds and then relaxing for 5 seconds. Repeat 20 times to strengthen your pelvic floor.

Cool Down (5 minutes)

1. **Spine Lengthening (3 minutes):** Sit upright and reach your hands overhead, stretching upward and holding for 10 seconds. Repeat 5 times to lengthen your spine.
2. **Deep Breathing (2 minutes):** Focus on slow, deep breaths, inhaling for 5 seconds and exhaling for 5 seconds. Repeat 10 times to end your session feeling relaxed.

Day 13: Enhanced Lower Body Strength

Warm-Up (5 minutes)

1. **Heel-Toe Taps (2 minutes):** Sit comfortably and alternately tap your heels and toes on the floor, holding each tap for 1 second. Continue for 2 minutes to warm up your lower legs.

2. **Seated Marching (3 minutes):** Lift your knees alternately, holding each lift for 2 seconds. Continue for 3 minutes to engage your lower body muscles.

Main Workout (15 minutes)

1. **Chair-Supported Tree Pose (5 minutes):** Stand behind your chair and place one foot on the opposite inner thigh. Hold for 20 seconds, then switch sides. Repeat 3 times per side to improve balance and strength.
2. **Seated Warrior II (5 minutes):** Sit on the edge of your chair and extend one leg out to the side. Stretch your arms out parallel to the floor and hold for 20 seconds. Switch sides and repeat 3 times per side to strengthen your legs and core.
3. **Seated Leg Lifts (5 minutes):** Lift one leg straight in front of you and hold for 5 seconds. Alternate legs and repeat 10 times per leg to strengthen your quadriceps.

Cool Down (5 minutes)

1. **Gentle Twists (3 minutes):** Sit and twist your torso to each side, holding each twist for 10 seconds. Repeat 6 times per side to stretch your back and sides.
2. **Deep Breathing (2 minutes):** Sit back, close your eyes, and focus on your breath. Inhale deeply for 5 seconds and exhale for 5 seconds. Repeat 10 times to relax.

Day 14: Upper Body and Core Integration

Warm-Up (5 minutes)

1. **Arm Reaches (3 minutes):** Sit and reach your arms up alternately, holding each reach for 3 seconds. Continue for 3 minutes to warm up your upper body.
2. **Torso Twists (2 minutes):** Twist your upper body to each side, holding each twist for 5 seconds. Repeat 5 times per side to loosen up your torso.

Main Workout (15 minutes)

1. **Seated Row (5 minutes):** Sit and pretend to row with both arms, squeezing your shoulder blades together. Hold each 'row' for 3 seconds and repeat 20 times to strengthen your back.

2. **Seated Belly Twist (5 minutes):** Twist your torso to one side with your hands on your shoulders, holding for 10 seconds. Switch sides and repeat 10 times per side to engage your core.
3. **Seated Knee Lifts (5 minutes):** Lift one knee toward your chest and hold for 5 seconds. Alternate knees and repeat 10 times per knee to strengthen your lower abs.

Cool Down (5 minutes)

1. **Arm and Shoulder Stretches (3 minutes):** Extend one arm across your body and hold it with your other hand, stretching for 10 seconds. Switch arms and repeat 3 times per arm to stretch your shoulders.
2. **Deep Breathing (2 minutes):** Sit back, close your eyes, and focus on your breath. Inhale deeply for 5 seconds and exhale for 5 seconds. Repeat 10 times to end your session feeling calm and refreshed.

Day 15: Focus on Breath and Movement

Warm-Up (5 minutes)

1. **Seated Arm Swings (3 minutes):** Sit and gently swing your arms from side to side, syncing the movement with your breathing. Continue for 3 minutes to get your blood flowing.
2. **Head Tilts (2 minutes):** Slowly tilt your head from side to side, holding each tilt for 5 seconds. Repeat 6 times on each side to release tension in your neck.

Main Workout (15 minutes)

1. **Seated Sun Salutations (7 minutes):** Flow through a series of seated yoga poses, coordinating your movements with your breath. Continue for 7 minutes to energize your body and mind.
2. **Chair Pigeon Pose (4 minutes):** While seated, place one ankle on the opposite knee and lean forward gently. Hold for 20 seconds on each side and repeat twice per side to stretch your hips.
3. **Seated Spinal Twist (4 minutes):** Twist your torso to one side and hold for 15 seconds. Switch sides and repeat 4 times per side to increase spinal flexibility.

Cool Down (5 minutes)

1. **Gentle Side Bends (3 minutes):** Reach one arm overhead and bend to the side, holding for 10 seconds. Repeat 3 times per side to stretch your sides.
2. **Meditation (2 minutes):** Sit quietly and focus on your breathing, allowing your mind to calm and relax.

Day 16: Gentle Strength Building

Warm-Up (5 minutes)

1. **Shoulder Rolls (3 minutes):** Roll your shoulders in a circular motion, 10 times forward and 10 times backward, to loosen up your shoulder joints.
2. **Neck Stretches (2 minutes):** Gently stretch your neck to each side, holding each stretch for 10 seconds. Repeat 3 times per side to ease neck tension.

Main Workout (15 minutes)

1. **Seated Leg Lifts (5 minutes):** Extend one leg at a time, holding it straight for 5 seconds before lowering slowly. Repeat 10 times per leg to strengthen your quadriceps.
2. **Seated Arm Raises (5 minutes):** Raise your arms to shoulder level and then overhead, holding each position for 2 seconds. Repeat 15 times to build shoulder strength.
3. **Seated Calf Raises (5 minutes):** Lift your heels off the ground and hold for 3 seconds before lowering. Repeat 20 times to strengthen your calves.

Cool Down (5 minutes)

1. **Seated Forward Bend (3 minutes):** Lean forward gently from your hips and reach toward your feet, holding the stretch for 15 seconds. Repeat 3 times to relax your back and hamstrings.
2. **Deep Breathing (2 minutes):** Sit comfortably and focus on deep breathing. Inhale for 5 seconds and exhale for 5 seconds. Repeat 10 times to end your session feeling calm and centered.

Day 17: Core and Posture

Warm-Up (5 minutes)

1. **Seated Cat-Cow (3 minutes):** Sit comfortably and alternate between arching your back (looking up) and rounding your back (tucking your chin). Sync your breath with each movement and repeat 10 times.
2. **Side Neck Stretches (2 minutes):** Gently tilt your head to each side, holding each stretch for 10 seconds. Repeat 5 times per side to loosen your neck muscles.

Main Workout (15 minutes)

1. **Seated Twist (5 minutes):** Sit up and rotate your torso to one side, holding for 15 seconds. Switch sides and repeat 6 times per side to enhance spinal flexibility.
2. **Chair Boat Pose (5 minutes):** Sit on the edge of your chair, lean back slightly, and lift your legs. Hold for 10 seconds and repeat 5 times to strengthen your core.
3. **Seated Forward Bend (5 minutes):** Lean forward from your hips and reach toward the ground, holding for 20 seconds. Repeat 3 times to stretch your lower back and hamstrings.

Cool Down (5 minutes)

1. **Overhead Stretch (3 minutes):** Reach your arms overhead and stretch upward, holding for 10 seconds. Repeat 3 times to lengthen your spine and improve posture.
2. **Deep Breathing (2 minutes):** Sit comfortably and focus on deep breathing. Inhale for 5 seconds and exhale for 5 seconds. Repeat 10 times to finish feeling relaxed.

Day 18: Gentle Cardio and Mobility

Warm-Up (5 minutes)

1. **Arm Circles (3 minutes):** Sit comfortably and perform large and small arm circles, spending 1 minute in each direction to warm up your shoulders.
2. **Seated Marching (2 minutes):** Lift your knees alternately, gradually increasing your pace to gently raise your heart rate. Continue for 2 minutes.

Main Workout (15 minutes)

1. **Seated March (5 minutes):** Lift each knee alternately as if you're marching. Hold each lift for 2 seconds and continue for 10-12 reps. Rest briefly and then repeat the march for a total of 32 times.
2. **Seated Bicycle (5 minutes):** Sit on the edge of your chair and perform a bicycle leg motion, mimicking pedaling. Continue for 5 minutes to engage your core and legs, resting for periods of 10-20 seconds when necessary.
3. **Ankle Crank (3 minutes)** Place one ankle on the opposite thigh. Hold your ankle with one hand and gently rotate it in a circular motion using your other hand. Do this 10 times in each direction, then switch legs. Repeat for 3 minutes, alternating legs.

Cool Down (5 minutes)

1. **Seated Leg Stretches (3 minutes):** Extend one leg and reach toward your toes, holding for 20 seconds. Switch your legs and repeat to stretch your hamstrings.
2. **Relaxation Breathing (2 minutes):** Sit comfortably and focus on relaxing each body part sequentially while breathing deeply. This helps to calm your mind and body.

Day 19: Gentle Cardio and Leg Strength

Warm-Up (5 minutes)

1. **Arm and Leg Coordination (3 minutes):** Sit comfortably and lift the opposite arm and leg simultaneously, holding for 2 seconds. Alternate sides and repeat 10 times on each side to warm up your body.
2. **Seated Twists (2 minutes):** Rotate your upper body gently from left to right, holding each twist for 5 seconds. Repeat 6 times on each side to loosen your spine.

Main Workout (15 minutes)

1. **Chair Lunge (5 minutes):** Stand behind a chair, holding onto the back for support, and step one foot back, keeping your front knee over your ankle. Lower your back knee toward the floor, then push through your front heel to return to the starting position. Repeat on both sides.

2. **Chair Squats (5 minutes):** Stand up from your chair and sit back down slowly, focusing on controlled movements. Repeat 10 times to strengthen your legs.
3. **Seated Toe Touches (5 minutes):** Extend your legs and reach toward your toes, holding the stretch for 10 seconds. Repeat 5 times to stretch your hamstrings.

Cool Down (5 minutes)

1. **Overhead Arm Stretch (3 minutes):** Reach your arms overhead and hold for 10 seconds. Release and repeat 5 times to stretch your upper body.
2. **Mindful Breathing (2 minutes):** Sit comfortably and breathe deeply, focusing on relaxing each part of your body.

Day 20: Upper Body Strength and Stability

Warm-Up (5 minutes)

1. **Shoulder and Neck Stretches (3 minutes):** Stretch your neck to each side and roll your shoulders, holding each stretch for 10 seconds to release tension.
2. **Wrist and Ankle Rotations (2 minutes):** Rotate your wrists and ankles in both directions 10 times each to warm up your joints.

Main Workout (15 minutes)

1. **Seated Warrior Poses (5 minutes):** Perform the Warrior II pose (sit on the edge of the chair with your feet on the ground, extend one leg out to the side, keeping the knee bent at a right angle, and stretch your arms out horizontally at shoulder height, gazing over your front hand) on each side, holding for 20 seconds. Repeat to strengthen your upper body and improve stability.
2. **Seated Shoulder Press (5 minutes):** Lift your arms to shoulder height and press overhead. Do 4-10 repetitions, rest, and repeat for 3 sets to build shoulder strength.
3. **Seated Camel Pose (5 minutes):** Lean back gently and hold for 5-10 seconds. Repeat 3-5 times, rest, and do 2 more sets to stretch your back and chest.

Cool Down (5 minutes)

1. **Seated Gentle Twists (3 minutes):** Twist your torso gently to each side, holding for 10 seconds. Repeat 6 times per side to relax your spine.

2. **Calming Breaths (2 minutes):** Inhale slowly for 5 seconds and exhale for 5 seconds. Repeat 10 times to finish your session feeling calm and centered.

Day 21: Integration and Relaxation

Warm-Up (5 minutes)

1. **Head Nods (3 minutes):** Sit and slowly nod your head up and down, then side to side. Hold each position for 5 seconds to ease any tension in your neck.
2. **Arm Stretches (2 minutes):** Stretch your arms out and across your body, holding each stretch for 10 seconds on each side to warm up your upper body.

Main Workout (15 minutes)

1. **Full Body Seated Stretches (7 minutes):** Flow through a sequence of stretches for your arms, legs, and torso. Hold each stretch for 10 seconds and enjoy the gentle movements.
2. **Seated Mountain Pose (4 minutes):** Sit up with your arms stretched overhead. Hold this pose for 10 seconds and repeat 6 times to enhance your posture and stability.
3. **Corpse Pose (4 minutes):** Sit comfortably in your chair with your feet flat on the floor, hands resting on your thighs or in your lap, and close your eyes. Focus on relaxing each part of your body from head to toe while taking slow, deep breaths, allowing yourself to fully unwind.

Cool Down (5 minutes)

1. **Gentle Seated Yoga Flow (3 minutes):** Move gently between seated poses, focusing on smooth transitions to calm your body and mind. *Example*: Start in a seated mountain pose with your back straight and arms resting by your sides, then slowly raise your arms overhead into a seated stretch. Transition smoothly into a seated forward bend by gently leaning forward from your hips, reaching towards your toes, and holding the stretch.
1. **Final Meditation (2 minutes):** Close your eyes, focus on your breath, and reflect on your 21-day journey. Think about how you can incorporate chair yoga into your daily routine moving forward.

21–DAY CHAIR YOGA CHALLENGE TRACKER

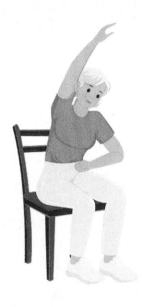

Day 1 ☐

Warmup
☐ Deep Breathing
☐ Neck Stretches

Main Workout
☐ Cat-Cow
☐ Side Stretch
☐ Flexing Foot Pose

Cool Down
☐ Deep Breathing (corpse pose)
☐ Seated Meditation

Day 2 ☐

Warmup
☐ Shoulder Rolls
☐ Arm Lifts

Main Workout
☐ Seated Twist
☐ Seated Eagle Arms
☐ Wrist & Finger Stretches

Cool Down
☐ Gentle Neck Rolls
☐ Arm Stretches

Day 3 ☐

Warmup
☐ Ankle Rolls
☐ Knee Lifts

Main Workout
☐ Seated Leg Lifts
☐ Ankle Stretches
☐ Chair Squats

Cool Down
☐ Leg & Calf Stretch
☐ Deep Breathing

Day 4 ☐

Warmup
☐ Side Bends
☐ Seated Marching

Main Workout
☐ Seated Pelvic Tilts
☐ Abdominal Bracing
☐ Seated Side Stretch

Cool Down
☐ Full Body Stretch
☐ Deep Breathing

Day 5 ☐

Warmup
☐ Toe Taps
☐ Heel Raises

Main Workout
☐ Single Leg Lifts
☐ Chair Plank
☐ Warrior Pose I

Cool Down
☐ Seated Forward Bend
☐ Deep Breathing

Day 6 ☐

Warmup
☐ Neck Tilts
☐ Shoulder Shrugs

Main Workout
☐ Cat-Cow Pose
☐ Mountain Forward Bend
☐ Seated twists

Cool Down
☐ Wrist & Finger Stretches
☐ Seated Meditation

Day 7 ☐

Warmup
☐ Gentle Neck Roll
☐ Shoulder Shrugs

Main Workout
☐ Breathing Exercises
☐ Seated twist/Side Stretch
☐ Seated Low Lunge

Cool Down
☐ Guided Relaxation
☐ Meditation

Week 1 Complete!

☐

Day 8

Warmup
- [ ] Arm Circles
- [ ] Shoulder Stretches

Main Workout
- [ ] Seated Row
- [ ] Arm Raises
- [ ] Tricep Stretches

Cool Down
- [ ] Neck Stretches
- [ ] Deep Breathing

Day 9

Warmup
- [ ] Knee Hugs
- [ ] Leg Swings

Main Workout
- [ ] Hamstring Stretch
- [ ] Flexing Foot Pose
- [ ] Seated Pigeon Pose

Cool Down
- [ ] Ankle Rolls
- [ ] Deep Breathing

Day 10

Warmup
- [ ] Seated Twists
- [ ] Side Bends

Main Workout
- [ ] Cat-Cow
- [ ] Gentle Backbends
- [ ] Spinal Twist

Cool Down
- [ ] Full Back Stretch
- [ ] Deep Breathing

Day 11

Warmup
- [ ] Arm & Leg Reaches
- [ ] Seated Twists

Main Workout
- [ ] Seated Forward Bend
- [ ] Seated Side Stretch
- [ ] Neck & Shoulder Rolls

Cool Down
- [ ] Full Body Relaxation
- [ ] Deep Breathing

Day 12

Warmup
- [ ] Pelvic Tilts
- [ ] Seated Marching

Main Workout
- [ ] Abdominal Twists
- [ ] Boat Pose
- [ ] Pelvic Floor Exercises

Cool Down
- [ ] Spine Lengthening
- [ ] Deep Breathing

Day 13

Warmup
- [ ] Heel-Toe Taps
- [ ] Seated Marching

Main Workout
- [ ] Tree Pose
- [ ] Seated Warrior II
- [ ] Seated Leg Lifts

Cool Down
- [ ] Gentle Twists
- [ ] Deep Breathing

Day 14

Warmup
- [ ] Arm Reaches
- [ ] Torso Twists

Main Workout
- [ ] Seated Row
- [ ] Seated Belly Twists
- [ ] Seated Knee Lifts

Cool Down
- [ ] Arm & Shoulder Stretches
- [ ] Deep Breathing

Week 2 Complete!

Day 15 ☐

Warmup
- ☐ Seated Arm Swings
- ☐ Head Tilts

Main Workout
- ☐ Seated Sun Salutations
- ☐ Chair Pigeon Pose
- ☐ Seated Spinal Twist

Cool Down
- ☐ Gentle Side Bend
- ☐ Meditation

Day 16 ☐

Warmup
- ☐ Shoulder Rolls
- ☐ Neck Stretches

Main Workout
- ☐ Seated Leg Lifts
- ☐ Seated Arm Raises
- ☐ Seated Calf Raises

Cool Down
- ☐ Seated Forward Bend
- ☐ Deep Breathing

Day 17 ☐

Warmup
- ☐ Seated Cat-Cow
- ☐ Seated Neck Stretches

Main Workout
- ☐ Seated Twist
- ☐ Chair Boat Pose
- ☐ Seated Forward Bend

Cool Down
- ☐ Overhead Stretch
- ☐ Deep Breathing

Day 18 ☐

Warmup
- ☐ Arm Circles
- ☐ Seated Marching

Main Workout
- ☐ Seated March
- ☐ Seated Bicycle
- ☐ Ankle Crank

Cool Down
- ☐ Seated Leg Stretches
- ☐ Relaxation Breathing

Day 19 ☐

Warmup
- ☐ Arm & Leg Coordination
- ☐ Seated Twists

Main Workout
- ☐ Chair Lunge
- ☐ Chair Squats
- ☐ Seated Toe Touches

Cool Down
- ☐ Overhead Arm Stretch
- ☐ Mindful Breathing

Day 20 ☐

Warmup
- ☐ Shoulder & Neck Stretches
- ☐ Wrist & Ankle Rotation

Main Workout
- ☐ Seated Warrior II
- ☐ Seated Shoulder Press
- ☐ Seated Camel Pose

Cool Down
- ☐ Seated Gentle Twists
- ☐ Calming Breaths

Day 21 ☐

Warmup
- ☐ Head Nods
- ☐ Arm Stretches

Main Workout
- ☐ Seated Stretches
- ☐ Mountain Pose
- ☐ Corpse Pose

Cool Down
- ☐ Seated Yoga Flow
- ☐ Final Meditation

21-Day Challenge Complete!

☐

How to Build Your Own Routine

You've completed the 21-day chair yoga challenge—congratulations! Now that you've experienced a variety of exercises and stretches, you have the tools to create your own personalized routine. Here's a guide to help you build a routine that suits your needs and preferences.

Best Practices for Creating Your Own Routine

1. **Focus on Exercises You Enjoyed:** Think back to the exercises that felt good and left you feeling energized and happy. These are the movements you'll want to include regularly.
2. **Choose Comfortable Stretches:** Include stretches where you felt a good, comfortable stretch and noticed improvements in your flexibility. These stretches will help you maintain and improve your range of motion.
3. **Incorporate Challenging Exercises:** Add in the exercises and poses that pushed you physically but where you also felt a sense of progress. These movements will help you build strength and endurance over time.
4. **Avoid Uncomfortable Movements:** Exclude any exercises that felt too uncomfortable or posed a risk of injury. Your routine should feel safe and sustainable.
5. **Consult with a Professional:** If you're unsure about certain exercises or want a more tailored routine, consider consulting with a yoga instructor or physical therapist. They can help you build a routine that aligns with your goals and any physical challenges you might have.
6. **Consider Your Goals:** Think about what you want to improve the most—whether it's flexibility, strength, balance, or relaxation. Focus on including exercises that target those areas.

Creating Your Routine

Here is a template that will help you craft a routine suited just right for you:

1. **Warm-Up (5-10 minutes):** Start with gentle movements to get your body ready. This could include arm circles, seated marching, or neck stretches.
2. **Main Workout (15-20 minutes):** Choose a mix of your favorite exercises and stretches.

3. **Cool Down (5-10 minutes):** End with calming movements to bring your heart rate down and relax your muscles. This might include gentle seated yoga flows or deep breathing exercises.

Remember, your routine is flexible and should evolve as you continue your yoga journey. Feel free to mix things up, try new exercises, and adjust as needed. The most important thing is that your routine feels good and supports your overall well-being.

As you continue to enjoy the benefits of chair yoga, it's important to remember that overall well-being involves more than just physical exercise. In the next chapter, we'll explore essential self-care practices for seniors, focusing on holistic approaches to maintain both your mental and physical health.

Chair Yoga Routines to Try
Morning Chair Yoga Routine

Let's start our day with some gentle movements to wake up our bodies and minds. This routine is perfect for getting your blood flowing and setting a positive tone for the day.

Warm-Up (5 minutes)

1. **Neck Rolls (1 minute):** Slowly roll your head in a circle, gently stretching your neck in one direction and then the other.
2. **Arm Circles (1 minute):** Extend your arms out to the sides and make small circles. Gradually make the circles bigger, then reverse the direction.
3. **Shoulder Rolls (1 minute):** Lift your shoulders to your ears, then roll them back and down.
4. **Seated Marches (1 minute):** Sit in a chair and lift your knees one at a time as if you're marching in place.
5. **Ankle Rolls (1 minute):** Lift one foot off the floor and roll your ankle in a circle. Do this for the other foot as well.

Main Workout

1. **Seated Mountain Pose (1 minute):** Sit up straight with your feet flat on the floor and hands resting on your thighs. Close your eyes and take deep breaths.

2. **Seated Cat-Cow Stretch (2 minutes):** Place your hands on your knees. Inhale as you arch your back and look up (Cow Pose), then exhale as you round your back and tuck your chin to your chest (Cat Pose). Repeat this flow.
3. **Seated Side Bend (1 minute each side):** Reach your right arm up and over your head, bending to the left. Hold, then switch to the other side.
4. **Seated Forward Bend (1 minute):** Inhale deeply, then exhale as you fold forward from your hips, reaching your hands towards your feet. Relax your head and neck, letting gravity do the work.
5. **Seated Twist (1 minute each side):** Place your right hand on the back of your chair and your left hand on your right knee. Inhale to sit straight, then exhale as you gently twist to the right. Hold for a minute, then switch to the other side.
6. **Seated Leg Raises (1 minute):** Sit back in your chair and lift one leg straight out in front of you, hold for a few seconds, then lower it. Alternate legs.
7. **Deep Breathing and Relaxation (2 minutes):** Finish your routine by closing your eyes and taking slow, deep breaths. Inhale through your nose, hold for a moment, then exhale through your mouth. Feel the calm and relaxation wash over you.

Evening Chair Yoga Routine

This routine is perfect for relaxing your body and mind before bedtime.

Warm-Up (4 Minutes)

1. **Seated Torso Circles (1 minute):** Sit comfortably and place your hands on your knees. Slowly circle your torso, leaning forward, to the side, back, and to the other side.
2. **Seated Cat-Cow Stretch (1 minute):** Place your hands on your knees. Inhale as you arch your back and look up (Cow Pose), then exhale as you round your back and tuck your chin to your chest (Cat Pose). Move gently and feel the soothing stretch.
3. **Arm Circles (1 minute):** Extend your arms to the sides and make small circles. Gradually increase the size of the circles, then reverse the direction.
4. **Shoulder Rolls (1 minute):** Lift your shoulders to your ears, then roll them back and down. Repeat.

Main Workout

1. **Seated Deep Breathing (3 minutes):** Close your eyes and place your hands on your belly. Inhale deeply through your nose, feeling your belly rise, then exhale slowly through your mouth. Focus on your breath.
2. **Seated Neck Stretches (2 minutes):** Gently tilt your head to the right, bringing your right ear toward your shoulder. Hold for a minute, then switch to the left side. Feel the gentle stretch along your neck.
3. **Seated Side Bend (2 minutes):** Reach your right arm up and over your head, bending to the left. Hold for a minute, enjoying the stretch along your side, then switch to the other side.
4. **Seated Twist (2 minutes):** Place your right hand on the back of your chair and your left hand on your right knee. Inhale to sit up, then exhale as you gently twist to the right. Hold, then switch to the other side.
5. **Seated Forward Bend (2 minutes):** Inhale deeply, then exhale as you fold forward from your hips, reaching your hands toward your feet. Relax your head and neck.
6. **Seated Cat-Cow Stretch (2 minutes):** Place your hands on your knees. Inhale as you arch your back and look up (Cow Pose), then exhale as you round your back and tuck your chin to your chest (Cat Pose). Repeat this gentle flow.

Flexibility and Mobility Chair Yoga Routine

This routine is perfect for loosening up those muscles and feeling more limber.

Warm-Up (6 Minutes)

1. **Seated Cat-Cow Stretch (2 minutes):** Start by placing your hands on your knees. Inhale as you arch your back and look up (Cow Pose), then exhale as you round your back and tuck your chin to your chest (Cat Pose). This movement will loosen up your back and abdominal muscles.
2. **Arm Overhead Stretches (1 minute each side):** Reach your right arm overhead and lean gently to the left, feeling a nice stretch along your side. Hold for a minute, then switch to the other side.
3. **Wrist and Finger Stretches (2 minutes):** Stretch out your fingers and wrists by extending your arms in front of you and gently pulling back on each finger. This prepares your hands and wrists for the flexibility work ahead.

Main Workout

1. **Seated Spinal Twist (2 minutes each side):** Sit up and place your right hand on the back of your chair and your left hand on your right knee. Inhale to lengthen your spine, then exhale as you twist to the right. Hold for two minutes, then switch to the other side.
2. **Seated Hip Opener (2 minutes each side):** Place your right ankle on your left knee and gently lean forward, feeling the stretch in your hip. Hold for two minutes, then switch legs.
3. **Chair Pigeon Pose (1 minute each side):** Similar to the hip opener, but deepen the stretch by leaning further forward. Hold for a minute on each side, enjoying the release in your hips.
4. **Forward Bend (2 minutes):** Extend your legs forward and reach toward your toes, stretching your hamstrings and lower back. Hold the stretch for 15-30 seconds, then release and repeat until you've stretched for a total of two minutes.
5. **Neck Stretch (30 seconds, rest, 30 more seconds):** Gently pull your head toward your right shoulder to stretch the left side of your neck. Hold for 30 seconds, rest, then repeat on the other side.
6. **Deep Breathing and Relaxation (3 minutes):** Finish your routine by closing your eyes and taking slow, deep breaths. Inhale deeply through your nose, hold for a moment, then exhale slowly through your mouth. Let the relaxation enhance your flexibility and mobility.

Balance and Stability Chair Yoga Routine

This sequence will help you feel more steady and secure.

Warm-Up (6 Minutes)

1. **Seated Toe and Heel Raises (2 minutes):** Alternate between lifting your toes and then your heels while seated.
2. **Seated Gentle Torso Twists (2 minutes):** Sit up and gently twist your torso to the left and then to the right to engage your core and warm up your spine.
3. **Shoulder Shrugs and Rolls (2 minutes):** Lift your shoulders toward your ears, then roll them back and down. Repeat.

Main Workout

1. **Seated Marching (2 minutes):** Simulate a marching motion while seated, lifting your knees alternately to engage your core and improve stability.
2. **Chair-Assisted Tree Pose (1 minute):** Place one foot on the opposite ankle or calf, using the chair for support. Hold, then switch legs. Do 3 reps for each leg.
3. **Chair Plank (1 minute):** Place both hands on the arms of the chair or the seat and hold your body in a plank position. This will engage your core and stabilize your upper body.
4. **Camel Pose Reps (15 seconds each with a short rest in between):** Sit on the edge of your chair with your feet flat on the ground. Place your hands on your lower back and gently arch your back, lifting your chest towards the ceiling. Hold for 15 seconds, then rest and repeat.
5. **Deep Breathing and Relaxation (3 minutes):** Finish your routine with deep, controlled breathing. Inhale deeply through your nose, hold for a moment, then exhale slowly through your mouth. Let this relaxation enhance your sense of balance and stability.

CHAPTER 10

SELF-CARE FOR SENIORS

"Self-care is not a waste of time. Self-care makes your use of time more sustainable."

—Jackie Viramontez

If you are not taking care of yourself off the chair, you won't see the results and recovery you hope for. This sentiment is echoed by many health professionals and fitness enthusiasts alike, and it holds especially true for seniors. To illustrate the importance of self-care and holistic health, let's look at the example of Jane Fonda [10]. Born in 1937 and in her 80s, this celebrity has shown the world that age is not a barrier to staying active and healthy. Her dedication to fitness began in the late 1970s and early 1980s, a time when she transformed not only her own life but also the fitness industry.

In the late 1970s, Jane released her first exercise video, "Jane Fonda's Workout" in 1982. This video became the highest-selling VHS of the time, making aerobics accessible to a broader audience. Her approach was straightforward and relatable, focusing on low-impact exercises that could be done at home. Her routines emphasized cardiovascular health, strength, and flexibility, making fitness enjoyable and attainable for people of all ages.

As Jane aged, her fitness philosophy evolved. She transitioned from high-intensity aerobics to more gentle forms of exercise that are easier on the joints. This included activities like yoga, stretching, and strength training. Her later videos and books reflected this shift, catering to an older demographic and promoting sustainable, long-term fitness practices.

Jane has always emphasized the importance of a holistic approach to health. She incorporates mindfulness and meditation into her routine, recognizing the connection between physical and mental well-being. Her fitness journey is not just about staying in shape. It's about fostering overall health and wellness.

Jane's journey is a testament to the power of exercise in enhancing quality of life, regardless of age. Through her example, she has shown that self-care can lead to a happier, healthier, and more fulfilling life.

What is Self-Care and Why is it Important?

Self-care is any action or practice we engage in regularly to maintain and improve our overall health and well-being. As we advance in age, the need for self-care becomes even more acute. Our bodies undergo various changes and recovery times from just day-to-day living can be longer. For seniors, practicing self-care means paying extra attention to factors like nutrition, hydration, and sleep, listening to our bodies, and making adjustments to our routines to meet our changing needs.

Self-care goes deeper than just catering to our physical bodies. It also involves activities that nourish our heart, mind, and spirit, which is the epitome of holistic health. Holistic health is an approach that considers the whole person, including physical, mental, emotional, and spiritual aspects, rather than just treating specific symptoms or conditions. It's about finding balance in all areas of life and recognizing how interconnected these areas are.

As we age, adopting a holistic approach to self-care makes a significant difference in our quality of life. We need to be proactive and intentional with our health practices. By integrating various forms of self-care into our daily routines, we can address the needs of our bodies, minds, and spirits, ensuring that we remain vibrant and healthy at every stage of life.

Practicing Holistic Self-Care as We Age

Physical Self-Care

As we age, our bodies require gentler yet consistent physical care in these forms:

Eating Healthy

A well-balanced diet is crucial for overall health. This means consuming a variety of foods that provide essential nutrients: plenty of fruits and vegetables, whole grains, lean proteins, and healthy fats. Avoiding processed foods is also important, as they often contain high levels of sugar, unhealthy fats, and preservatives. Here are some common processed foods to steer clear of:

- Packaged snacks (chips, cookies)
- Sugary drinks (sodas, energy drinks)
- Processed meats (hot dogs, sausages)
- Fast food
- Ready-made meals

Staying Hydrated

Drinking enough water throughout the day is essential, especially before and after activities like chair yoga. Proper hydration helps maintain energy levels, supports digestion, and keeps our joints lubricated. Aim for at least 8 glasses of water a day, but remember that individual needs can vary based on factors like activity level and climate.

Creating a Workout Routine

Working out regularly is key to staying healthy as we age. Creating a routine and sticking to it helps build strength and endurance over time. If you're new to exercise or looking for guidance, the routines provided in this book will help you get started.

Prioritizing Sleep

Sleep is necessary for proper recovery and overall health. As we sleep, our bodies repair tissues, consolidate memories, and regulate various functions. Here are some tips to ensure you get adequate rest:

- **Maintain a regular sleep schedule:** Go to bed and wake up at the same time every day.
- **Create a bedtime routine:** Develop calming habits before bed, such as reading or taking a warm bath.
- **Optimize your sleep environment:** Ensure your bedroom is dark, quiet, and cool.
- **Limit screen time before bed:** Avoid using electronic devices at least an hour before bedtime.

Mental and Emotional Self-Care

Mental and emotional well-being are equally important as physical health. Caring for your heart and mind has a variety of benefits like:

- Stress reduction
- Improved mental clarity
- Emotional resilience
- Better relationships
- Increased happiness
- Enhanced self-awareness

Here are a few activities that will keep your heart and mind nimble:

Taking Time to Relax

Taking time to relax is essential for maintaining mental and emotional health. Relaxation helps reduce stress, improve mood, and promote overall well-being. Whether it's a quiet moment with a cup of tea, a leisurely walk in nature, or simply sitting in silence, find time to unwind.

Journaling

Journaling is a powerful emotional self-care tool. Writing about what you're grateful for helps shift focus to the positive aspects of life, fostering a sense of contentment. Additionally, journaling about your goals and dreams, a practice known as future manifesting, can provide clarity and motivation.

Connecting with Friends and Family

Spending time with loved ones is a vital component of emotional well-being. Regularly connecting with friends and family provides a sense of belonging and support. Whether it's through phone calls, video chats, or in-person visits, maintaining these relationships can significantly boost your mood and reduce feelings of loneliness.

While spending time with friends and family is incredibly important, there are many other ways you can expand your social circles and enrich your life:

Join a Club or Group

Joining a club or group that aligns with your interests is a fantastic way to meet new people. Whether it's a book club, gardening group, or walking club, these gatherings provide regular opportunities to socialize and share common passions.

Participate in Community Events

Local community centers often host events and activities specifically designed for seniors. These can include dance nights, art classes, or holiday celebrations. Participating in these events can help you meet people in your area and build new friendships.

Volunteer

Volunteering is a meaningful way to connect with others while giving back to your community. Many organizations, such as hospitals, schools, and charities, welcome the help of volunteers. This can lead to meeting like-minded individuals and forming lasting bonds.

Attend Senior Meetups

Meetup.com and similar platforms offer various groups and events tailored to seniors. From hiking trips to movie nights, there are many activities where you can meet new people and enjoy shared experiences.

Engage in Online Communities

The internet offers numerous platforms where seniors can socialize. From Facebook groups to forums and virtual classes, online communities provide a space to connect with others without leaving home. This can be especially beneficial for those with mobility issues or who live in remote areas.

Explore Hobbies

Pursuing hobbies like knitting, painting, or playing music in a group setting can be both enjoyable and social. Hobby groups or workshops provide a relaxed atmosphere to meet people with similar interests.

Pet Ownership and Animal Therapy Groups

Pets can be great companions, and joining pet-focused groups or participating in animal therapy sessions can help you meet other pet owners and animal lovers. This shared interest can be a great foundation for building new friendships.

Learning Something New

Keeping your brain active by learning something new can greatly benefit your mental health. Whether it's picking up a new hobby, taking an online course, or exploring a new topic, continuous learning helps keep the mind sharp and engaged. It's a fun and rewarding way to challenge yourself and discover new interests.

Spiritual Self-Care

Spirituality can provide a sense of purpose and connection to something greater than oneself, offering a profound sense of peace and fulfillment. Nurturing your spirit doesn't have to be complicated or even connected to a religious belief. It can be as simple as engaging in activities that resonate with you on a deeper level. Spirituality is a personal journey, and finding what resonates with you is key to enhancing your overall well-being.

Religious Practices

For many, spirituality is closely tied to religious practices. Attending services, participating in community activities, or simply reading religious texts can provide comfort and a sense of belonging. These practices often offer guidance, support, and a deeper connection to a higher power.

Meditation

Meditation is a powerful tool for nurturing the spirit. It involves focusing the mind and achieving a state of calm and clarity. Here are some tips for getting started:

- **Find a quiet space:** Choose a place where you won't be disturbed.
- **Set a time:** Start with just a few minutes each day and gradually increase.
- **Focus on your breath:** Pay attention to your breathing, letting thoughts come and go without judgment.
- **Use guided meditations:** There are many apps and online resources to help guide you through the process.

Time Spent in Nature

Nature has a remarkable ability to rejuvenate the spirit. Spending time outdoors, whether it's a walk in the park, a hike in the mountains, or simply sitting by a lake, can help you feel more connected to the world around you. Here are some ideas:

- **Take daily walks:** Even a short walk can clear your mind and lift your spirits.
- **Gardening:** Connecting with the earth and watching plants grow can be incredibly fulfilling.
- **Mindful observation:** Take a moment to sit quietly and observe the natural world around you, noticing the sounds, sights, and smells.

Art and Creativity

Engaging in creative activities like painting, writing, or music can be a profound form of spiritual expression, offering a unique way to connect with your inner self and the world around you. These activities provide an outlet for emotions, thoughts, and experiences that might be difficult to express otherwise. Whether it's the rhythmic brushstrokes on a canvas, the flow of words on a page, or the harmonious notes of a musical piece, creativity allows for a deep and personal exploration of our inner landscapes. This form of expression can be meditative, providing a sense of peace and fulfillment as we lose ourselves in the creative process. Moreover, sharing our art with others can foster a sense of community and connection, further enriching our spiritual journey. By engaging in creative pursuits, we not only nurture our souls but also contribute to a vibrant and expressive life, enhancing our overall well-being.

Implementing a Holistic Health Routine

To create a self-care routine that supports holistic health, start by identifying the activities that you enjoy and that make you feel good. Reflect on the exercises that felt comfortable and beneficial during your chair yoga sessions. Consider incorporating those into your daily routine along with other self-care practices that address your mental, emotional, and spiritual needs.

For example, you might start your day with a gentle yoga session, followed by a nutritious breakfast. Later, engage in a mentally stimulating activity like reading or solving puzzles. Ensure you make time for social interactions, whether through a phone call, a visit with friends, or participating in community events. Finally, include moments of reflection or meditation to nurture your spiritual health.

By taking care of your body, mind, and spirit, you can achieve a state of well-being that supports your full potential.

CONCLUSION

"Yoga is not about touching your toes. It is what you learn on the way down."

– Jigar Gor

As we wrap up our journey into chair yoga, it's essential to reflect on the impact this practice can have on our lives, especially as we age. For seniors over 60, chair yoga isn't just about staying active. It extends to embracing a holistic approach to wellness that nurtures the body, mind, and spirit. Let's revisit the key benefits and the transformative potential of integrating chair yoga into your daily routine.

A Gateway to Physical Wellness

Chair yoga offers a gentle yet effective way to maintain and improve physical health. The exercises are designed to enhance flexibility, strength, and balance without putting undue stress on the joints. This is particularly important as we age and our bodies require more thoughtful care to stay functional and resilient.

By incorporating chair yoga into your routine, you can experience:

- **Improved Mobility:** Regular practice helps keep your joints flexible, reducing stiffness and improving overall mobility.

- **Enhanced Strength:** Even simple chair yoga poses can help build muscle strength, support better posture, and reduce the risk of falls.
- **Better Balance:** Balance-focused exercises can enhance stability, which is crucial for preventing injuries in everyday activities.

Nurturing Mental and Emotional Health

Beyond the physical benefits, chair yoga is a powerful tool for mental and emotional well-being. The mindful nature of the practice encourages a deeper connection with yourself, promoting a sense of calm and clarity.

Engaging in chair yoga can help you:

- **Reduce Stress:** Deep breathing and gentle movements help activate the relaxation response, reducing stress and anxiety.
- **Enhance Mental Clarity:** The focus required for yoga helps keep your mind sharp, improving concentration and cognitive function.
- **Boost Emotional Resilience:** The meditative aspects of chair yoga foster a sense of peace and emotional balance, helping you navigate the ups and downs of life with greater ease.

Building a Supportive Community

One of the beautiful aspects of chair yoga is its potential to bring people together. Whether you join a local class or participate in online sessions, the sense of community and support can be incredibly enriching. Sharing your yoga journey with others can provide motivation, encouragement, and a sense of belonging.

Practical Tips for Continuing Your Practice

As you move forward with chair yoga, here are some practical tips to keep in mind:

- **Consistency is Key:** Aim to practice regularly, even if it's just for a few minutes each day. Consistency will yield the best results over time.

- **Listen to Your Body:** Pay attention to how your body feels during and after each session. Modify poses as needed to suit your comfort level and physical capabilities.
- **Explore and Adapt:** Don't be afraid to explore different styles and approaches to chair yoga. Adapt the practice to meet your unique needs and preferences.
- **Combine with Other Wellness Practices:** Integrate chair yoga with other healthy habits, such as proper nutrition, hydration, and adequate sleep, for a holistic approach to wellness.

Embrace the Journey

Chair yoga is more than just an exercise. It's a journey toward greater self-awareness and well-being. It's about honoring your body's capabilities and limitations, celebrating your progress, and nurturing your overall health.

As you continue this journey, remember that every pose, every breath, and every moment of mindfulness contributes to a healthier, happier you. Embrace chair yoga as a lifelong practice that evolves with you, providing support and enrichment through every stage of life. Share this book with another senior who can benefit from it, or leave a review of your experience with these words, and together, we can build a thriving aging community.

In conclusion, chair yoga offers a gentle, accessible, and profoundly beneficial way to stay active and healthy after 60. It empowers you to take charge of your well-being, fostering physical vitality, mental clarity, and emotional peace. So, sit in your chair, take a deep breath, and let the journey of chair yoga guide you to a vibrant and fulfilling life.

Thank you for reading!

If you havent already, I would greatly appreciate it if you could leave your feedback! As a small, independent publisher it really does wonders for the book and allows me to make more resources for you.

To leave your feedback:

- Open your camera app
- Point your mobile device at the QR code below
- The review page will appear in your web browser

You can also leave your feedback under your Amazon orders page.

Thank you!

REFERENCE

1. *Meditation and yoga can modulate brain mechanisms that affect behavior and Anxiety-A modern scientific perspective.* (2015). PubMed Central (PMC). https://www.ncbi.nlm.nih.gov/pmc/articles/PMC4769029/

2. *Perception of subtle energy "Prana", and its effects during Biofield practices: A qualitative meta-synthesis.* (2023, January). PubMed Central (PMC). https://www.ncbi.nlm.nih.gov/pmc/articles/PMC10498708/

3. Lindberg, S. *What are chakras? Meaning, location, and how to unblock them.* Healthline. https://www.healthline.com/health/what-are-chakras

4. *The surprising benefits of chair yoga.* Kripalu. https://kripalu.org/resources/surprising-benefits-chair-yoga

5. Development, B. (2022, January 19). *Great benefits of chair yoga for seniors.* Aston Gardens. https://www.astongardens.com/senior-living-blog/great-benefits-of-chair-yoga-for-seniors/

6. WebMD Editorial Contributors. (2021, April 9). *What is Breathwork?* WebMD. https://www.webmd.com/balance/what-is-breathwork

7. Cole, R. (2021, December 8). *Diaphragmatic breathing: The best way to breathe to advance your yoga practice.* Yoga Journal. https://www.yogajournal.com/practice/energetics/pranayama/your-best-breath/

8. *How breath-control can change your life: A systematic review on psycho-physiological correlates of slow breathing.* (2018). PubMed Central (PMC). https://www.ncbi.nlm.nih.gov/pmc/articles/PMC6137615/

9. *Pursed-lip breathing - StatPearls - NCBI bookshelf.* (2023, July 25). National Center for Biotechnology Information. https://www.ncbi.nlm.nih.gov/books/NBK545289/

10. *Jane Fonda.* (1998, July 20). Encyclopedia Britannica. https://www.britannica.com/biography/Jane-Fonda

Made in the USA
Coppell, TX
12 November 2024

40072974R00077